Pathological Demand Avoidance Syndrome
My Daughter is Not Naughty

of related interest

**Understanding Pathological Demand
Avoidance Syndrome in Children**
A Guide for Parents, Teachers and Other Professionals
Phil Christie, Margaret Duncan, Ruth Fidler and Zara Healy
Part of the JKP Essentials series
ISBN 978 1 84905 074 6
eISBN 978 0 85700 253 2

Can I tell you about Pathological Demand Avoidance Syndrome?
A guide for friends, family and professionals
Ruth Fidler and Phil Christie
Part of the Can I tell you about...? series
ISBN 978 1 84905 513 0
eISBN 978 0 85700 929 6

Pathological Demand Avoidance Syndrome

My Daughter is Not Naughty

JANE ALISON SHERWIN

Foreword and Introduction by Phil Christie

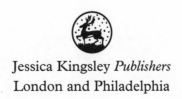

Jessica Kingsley *Publishers*
London and Philadelphia

First published in 2015
by Jessica Kingsley Publishers
73 Collier Street
London N1 9BE, UK
and
400 Market Street, Suite 400
Philadelphia, PA 19106, USA

www.jkp.com

Library of Congress Cataloging in Publication Data
A CIP catalog record for this book is available from the Library of Congress

British Library Cataloguing in Publication Data
A CIP catalogue record for this book is available from the British Library

ISBN 978 1 84905 614 4
eISBN 978 1 78450 085 6

Printed and bound in Great Britain

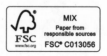

MIX
Paper from
responsible sources
FSC® C013056

I would like to dedicate this book to my wonderful daughter Mollie who has taught me compassion, patience, true empathy, courage and strength. The numerous battles that you face with humour, tenacity and resilience on a daily basis, to fit into a world that doesn't understand you, have truly inspired me. I hope that by allowing me to share your story, you will help and inspire those who will follow in your footsteps.

All my love and thank you Mollie Bear.

Mum

xxx

Contents

Foreword and Introduction

Pathological Demand Avoidance (PDA) was a term first used by Professor Elizabeth Newson in the 1980s. The initial descriptions of this profile were introduced in a series of lectures, presentations and papers that described a gradually developing understanding of a group of children who had been referred for diagnostic assessment at the clinic she led at the Child Development Research Unit at The University of Nottingham. Most of the children referred to the clinic were complex and unusual in their developmental profile, and many reminded the referring professionals of children with autism or Asperger's syndrome. At the same time, though, they were often seen as atypical in some way.

Newson and her colleagues felt increasingly dissatisfied with the description of 'atypical autism', feeling that it was not particularly helpful in removing the confusion that was often felt by parents and teachers who were struggling to gain greater insight into the child's behaviour. As time went by, it became apparent that while these children were atypical of those with autism or Asperger's syndrome, they were similar to each other in some very important ways. The central feature that was characteristic of all the children was 'an obsessional avoidance of the ordinary demands of everyday life' (Newson, Le Maréchal and David 2003).

This was combined with sufficient social understanding and sociability to enable the child to be 'socially manipulative' in their avoidance.

The full set of diagnostic criteria that Newson set out is reproduced in the first chapter of this book. Newson proposed that PDA should be seen as a separate syndrome within the pervasive developmental disorders, which was the recognised category used within the versions of the psychiatric classification systems at the time (ICD-10 put forward by the World Health Organization and DSM-IV by the American Psychiatric Association).

Newson's work on PDA attracted great interest, as well as a degree of controversy. The overriding reason for the interest has been the strong sense of recognition, expressed by both parents and professionals, of the behavioural profile that she so clearly described. Parents in particular recounted a 'light-bulb moment' on reading the accounts and a feeling that they were, at last, hearing a description that seemed to make sense of their child. The controversy that arose was about whether PDA existed as a separate syndrome within the pervasive developmental disorders or whether the behaviours could be explained within other diagnostic categories.

The accounts of PDA also resonated with a large number of teachers and other professionals who were finding that many of the tried and tested 'autism strategies' were proving less effective for children with the PDA profile. Newson and colleagues at Sutherland House School led the way in producing the first 'Education and Handling Guidelines' that promoted an approach based on being less directive and more flexible than the more structured methods usually advocated for children with autism. These guidelines have since been rewritten and adopted as part of the National Autism Standards, published by the Autism Education Trust (2012).

In the years following Newson *et al.*'s 2003 publication, the first paper on PDA to appear in a peer reviewed journal, it became apparent that the term 'autism spectrum disorder' (ASD) was being used interchangeably with pervasive developmental disorder. In fact, the National Autism Plan for Children (National Initiative for Autism: Screening and Assessment 2003) talked about the term ASD 'broadly coinciding with the term Pervasive Developmental Disorder'. The more recently published National Institute for Health and Care Excellence (NICE) guidelines on ASD, 'Autism Diagnosis in Children and Young People: Recognition, Referral and Diagnosis of Children and Young People on the Autism Spectrum' (National Institute for Health and Care Excellence 2011) described the two terms as being 'synonymous'.

The importance of this is that it is now increasingly recognised that PDA is best understood as being part of the autism spectrum or one of the autism spectrum conditions. This view was endorsed when the National Autistic Society (NAS) published an article about PDA in its magazine, *Communication*, (National Autistic Society 2009) and later updated its website to include information about the condition.

In 2011 the NAS and NORSACA worked collaboratively to hold the first national conference on PDA, which included presentations covering research, diagnosis, education and family support needs. At this conference, Francesca Happé, Professor of Cognitive Neuroscience at the Institute of Psychiatry, talked about the quality and detail of the clinical accounts of PDA and the strong recognition factor amongst parents and teachers. She went on to say that there was a real need to underpin this with empirical research. Liz O'Nions, working with Francesca Happé, Essie Viding and others, has carried out a number of studies over the last three years that have culminated in two articles being published in 2013: one in the *Journal of Child Psychology and Psychiatry* (O'Nions *et al.* 2013a) and another in *Autism: The International Journal of Research and Practice* (O'Nions *et al.* 2013b). The first of these describes the development and preliminary validation of the Extreme Demand Avoidance Questionnaire (EDA-Q), which has the potential to quantify PDA traits to assist in the identification and differentiation of this group for further research. Ultimately, this will enhance our understanding and clinical practice.

Knowledge and understanding of PDA is still at an early stage, but there are exciting developments happening in diagnostic understanding, greater awareness of successful educational approaches and the perspective that is now being gained from further research. All of these coming together provides an opportunity for wider recognition of the condition, as well as better understanding and support for individuals with PDA and their families.

Jane Sherwin's book, the account of the mother of Mollie, a ten-year-old girl with PDA, will add to that knowledge by highlighting the perspective of a parent, as well as giving fascinating glimpses into how the world seems from Mollie's point of view. It gives a moving and detailed account of 'one family's journey' covering Mollie's early history, the period leading up to and following her diagnosis and the family's experience within the educational system until they made the decision that it was in Mollie's best interests for her to be home-schooled. The book describes the frustrations and difficulties faced in their relationship with some professionals, in getting Mollie's needs understood and trying to obtain appropriate support.

This will be familiar to many other families. It also explains the stresses placed on the whole family by aspects of Mollie's behaviour, the imaginative strategies they have developed to reduce Mollie's anxiety and the ways in which they have adapted in order to accommodate her complex needs. Jane doesn't shy away from covering difficult topics in what she says is 'a raw, real and honest account', recounting the many challenges they have faced and the enormous impact of Mollie's condition on their lives. She also gives a host of useful strategies, reflections and tales of lighter moments and of Mollie's 'endearing side'.

The book is a unique account. PDA is best understood as part of the autism spectrum and, as such, it affects individuals to a greater or lesser extent and in different ways according to the severity of the condition and individual circumstances and characteristics. The level of Mollie's anxiety and the intensity of her outbursts represent an 'extreme presentation of PDA'. Jane is also keen to point out that some of her choices have been deeply personal, especially regarding Mollie's education and the decision to take her out of the school system. At the same time, many aspects of the account will resonate with other families' experiences. Parents and professionals alike will greatly benefit from reflecting on these experiences, trying to understand the world from Mollie's point of view and the helpful advice on strategies to deal with everyday problems.

Phil Christie
Consultant Child Psychologist, the Elizabeth Newson Centre

Acknowledgements

I'd like to express my gratitude to:

- The most wonderful, supportive, non-judgemental, self-sacrificing and loving parents that any daughter could possibly wish for. Your never-ending love and support has carried me through the darkest of times. Your acceptance of your granddaughter's condition and the continued love and adjustments that you made for her really have made all of the difference.

- Lee, I love you with all of my heart and the fact that our marriage has grown stronger through this very challenging journey is a testament to the concrete that holds us together.

- Jake, I could not wish for a more perfect, patient and accepting son, and my love for you knows no bounds. You have, without a single moan, consistently taken a back seat while we had to throw all of our energies into raising your sister.

- Marisha, for being completely thrown in at the deep end and having to continue to run our business, with only a few years' experience under your belt, when I had to leave to dedicate my time to Mollie.

- Brian, my father-in-law, you continued working well into your seventies to keep the business afloat and to support us during periods when Lee was unable to dedicate himself to work.

- Ann, thank you, you are a true friend to Mollie and also a great support to me. Your dedication, genuine affection and sense of fun have been so important for Mollie's progress.

- Neville Starnes, a fellow parent and commitee member of the PDA Society, you have helped me enormously to understand my daughter and I will always be grateful to you for sharing your knowledge, time and wisdom with me.

- Eric Page (educational psychologist), who gave me unwavering support throughout our journey and was an instrumental part in helping me secure understanding and support for Mollie in her education.

- Sue, for your wonderful observation skills and support, recognising autism spectrum disorder (ASD) traits in Mollie and the help that you offered Mollie in her education. Your natural affection for my daughter and her quirks was very much appreciated and welcomed.

- D. Clarke, Karen, Sarah, Lauren, Jo and Caroline, you all worked tirelessly to offer Mollie the best chance possible in her second school placement, and your dedication and respect were greatly appreciated.

- Sarah, Jonathan and Dan – Mollie's wonderful Outreach Team – and Debbie – Mollie's social work assistant, you believed in, accommodated and advocated for

Mollie. Sarah, you were a true lifesaver on more than one occasion and one of nicest and most caring people who I have ever met. I owe you so much for the years that you supported me and Mollie.

- Professor Elizabeth Newson, for discovering this unique group of individuals and working tirelessly in the field to ensure that this subgroup was rightfully recognised.

- Phil Christie, for continuing the work of Professor Elizabeth Newson and increasingly pushing Pathological Demand Avoidance (PDA) to the forefront of professional discussions.

- The PDA Society, for the huge help and support that your forum offered me way back when there was so little information about PDA on the internet and for the continued work that you do now.

- The 'PDA Army', who inhabit various support groups, forums and Facebook pages online. Without each other I really don't know how many of us would get through the daily trials and tribulations. Special thanks to Graeme for the personal work that you have done promoting and raising the profile of PDA online.

Part 1

The Early Years

1

The Key Diagnostic Features of PDA

The purpose of this book is to share my personal experience of living with a child with Pathological Demand Avoidance (PDA) to attempt to convey just how debilitating and complex a condition this is, both for the child and for their family. This book will be a very raw, real and honest account of our lives and the challenges that we have faced in coming to terms with and adjusting our lives to living with our daughter who was diagnosed with PDA at the Elizabeth Newson Centre when she was seven years old. However, I am also hopeful that our story can offer a small ray of light to many families by showing the positive progress that we have made so far.

By sharing our journey, I am hopeful that I may also enlighten many professionals about the fact that PDA is a very real condition, which is not caused by poor or inconsistent parenting and cannot be adequately explained by current diagnostic labels.

Before I begin to tell you about our personal journey, it is important to look at the key diagnostic features of PDA. It is important to bear in mind that the extreme, confusing and challenging behaviour is often the result of anxiety, frustration and confusion due to the individual's very complex difficulties associated with social understanding, social interaction, social communication and emotional problems to name but a few.

Elizabeth Newson revised and refined her descriptions of the PDA profile as her research and clinical understanding grew. This is the third revision of the criteria published by the Elizabeth Newson Centre in 2002 and subsequently included in the first peer-reviewed article of PDA in the *Archives of Diseases in Childhood* (Newson *et al.* 2003).

Key features of PDA

1. *Passive early history in first year:* Often the child doesn't reach, drops toys, 'just watches'; often delayed milestones. As more is expected of him/her, child becomes 'actively passive', that is, strongly objects to normal demands, resists. A few children actively resist from the start; everything is on own terms. Parents tend to adapt so completely that they are unprepared for the extent of failure once child is subjected to ordinary group demands of nursery or school; they realise child needs 'velvet gloves' but don't perceive as abnormal. Professionals see child as puzzling but normal at first.

2. *Continues to resist and avoid ordinary demands of life:* Seems to feel under intolerable pressure from normal expectations of young children; devotes self to actively avoiding these. Demand avoidance may seem the greatest social and cognitive skill and most obsessional preoccupation. As language develops, strategies of avoidance are essentially socially manipulative, often adapted to adult involved; they may include:

- distracting adult: 'Look out of the window!', 'I've got you a flower!', 'I love your necklace!', 'I'm going to be sick', 'Bollocks! – I said bollocks!'

- acknowledging demand but excusing self: 'I'm sorry, but I can't', 'I'm afraid I've got to do this first', 'I'd rather do this', 'I don't have to, you can't make me', 'You do it, and I'll…', 'Mummy wouldn't like me to'

- physically incapacitating self: hides under table, curls up in corner, goes limp, dissolves in tears, drops everything, seems unable to look in direction of task (though retains eye contact), removes clothes or glasses, 'I'm too hot', 'I'm too tired', 'It's too late now', 'I'm handicapped', 'I'm going blind/deaf', 'My hands have gone flat'

- withdrawing into fantasy, doll play, animal play: talks only to doll or to inanimate objects, appeals to doll: 'My girls won't let me do that', 'My teddy doesn't like this game', 'But I'm a tractor, tractors don't have hands', growls, bites

- reducing meaningful conversation: bombards adult with speech (or other noises, e.g. humming) to drown out demands, mimics purposefully, refuses to speak

- (as last resort) outbursts, screaming, hitting, kicking; best construed as a panic attack.

3. *Surface sociability, but apparent lack of sense of social identity, pride or shame:* At first sight, normally sociable (has enough empathy to manipulate adults as shown in item 2), but ambiguous (see item 4) and without depth. No negotiation with other children, doesn't identify with children as a category: the question 'Does she know she's a child?' makes sense to parents, who recognise this as a major problem. Wants other children

to admire, but usually shocks them by complete lack of boundaries. No sense of responsibility, not concerned with what is 'fitting to her age' (might pick fight with toddler). Despite social awareness, behaviour is uninhibited, for example, unprovoked aggression, extreme giggling/inappropriate laughter or kicking/screaming in shop or classroom. Prefers adults but doesn't recognise their status. Seems very naughty, but parents say 'not naughty but confused' and 'It's not that she can't or won't, but she *can't help won't* – parents at a loss, as are others. Praise, reward, reproof and punishment ineffective; behavioural approaches fail.

4. *Liability of mood, impulsive, led by need to control:* Switches from cuddling to thumping for no obvious reason, or both at once ('I hate you' while hugging, nipping while handholding). Very impetuous, has to follow impulse. Switching of mood may be response to perceived pressure; goes 'over the top' in protest or in fear reaction, or even in affection; emotions may seem like an 'act'. Activity must be on child's terms; can change mind in an instant if suspects someone else is exerting control. May apologise but reoffend at once, or totally deny the obvious. Teachers need great variety of strategies, not rule-based: novelty helps.

5. *Comfortable in role play and pretending:* Some appear to lose touch with reality. May take over second-hand roles as a convenient 'way of being', that is, coping strategy. Many behave to other children like the teacher (thus seem bossy); may mimic and extend styles to suit mood, or to control events or people. Parents often confused about 'who he really is'. May take charge of assessment in role of psychologist, or using puppets, which helps co-operation; may adopt

style of baby or of video character. Role play of 'good person' may help in school, but may divert attention from underachievement. Enjoys dolls/toy animals/domestic play. Copes with normal conventions of shared pretending. Indirect instruction helps.

6. *Language delay, seems result of passivity:* Good degree of catch-up, often sudden. Pragmatics not deeply disordered, good eye contact (sometimes over-strong); social timing fair except when interrupted by avoidance; facial expression usually normal or over-vivacious. However, speech content usually odd or bizarre, even discounting demand-avoidant speech. Social mimicry more common than video mimicry; brief echoing in some. Repetitive questions used for distraction, but may signal panic.

7. *Obsessive behaviour:* Much or most of the behaviour described is carried out in an obsessive way, especially demand avoidance; as a result, most children show very low level achievement in school because motivation to avoid demands is so sustained and because the child knows no boundaries to avoidance. Other obsessions tend to be social, that is, to do with people and their characteristics; some obsessionally blame or harass people they don't like or are overpowering in their liking for certain people; children may target other individual children.

8. *Neurological involvement:* Soft neurological signs are seen in the form of clumsiness and physical awkwardness; crawling late or absent in more than half. Some have absences, fits or episodic dyscontrol. Not enough hard evidence as yet.

2

The Early Warning Signs

Mollie Aged Six Months to Three Years

On 12 October my little bundle of joy, Mollie, made her entry into this world. My love for her was instantaneous and we shared an immediate bond. She was an absolute dream of a baby because she cried very little and slept for hours at a time. When she was awake she did need constant attention, but as long as this was provided, she was content and happy.

At approximately 18 months old Mollie became very difficult, which we put down to the 'terrible twos'. We had no concerns at this stage, because we simply saw these difficulties, although they were extreme, as typical behaviour for a nearly-two-year-old child.

My only yardstick for childhood development was my son, who was seven years old at that time. I had always found him to be very different to his peers, but I had been unable to get anyone of a professional standing to actually take my concerns seriously. It was even implied, on more than one occasion, that his difficulties were down to my parenting. He had always displayed challenging behaviour, had massive meltdowns over the smallest and most minor of things and had huge difficulty in simply dealing with the day-to-day occurrences of life. It wasn't until he was 14 years old that he would finally be diagnosed with Asperger's syndrome by a very experienced and well-respected clinician.

However, during this period of Mollie's development I was completely unaware of the fact that my seven-year-old son had Asperger's. I had been told by health professionals time and time again that he was a 'typical' child and so, when Mollie's behaviours began to replicate his, I naturally assumed that her challenging behaviours were 'typical' too.

However, unlike her brother who was extremely quiet and introverted, often appeared sad, hardly spoke and was cripplingly shy, Mollie was the polar opposite. She was extremely outgoing, bundles of fun, confident and a real extrovert. Everyone who met her instantly fell in love with her quirky and endearing character, which did help to balance out the newly emerging and more challenging side of her character.

I suppose that when I look back, we had the same difficulties as many other parents but ours simply appeared to be cranked up to the maximum at all times and were far more extreme compared with those of a typically developing child. Meltdowns would last forever, and everything and anything was a source of avoidance, refusal and pushing boundaries to the edge.

Simply getting dressed, for example, was a power battle that caused huge stress for all involved. There would be a stint on the naughty step between each layer of clothing. This would be very frustrating if you had to be somewhere for a certain time. The naughty step, despite my continual use of this method of control, did not cause or help Mollie to modify her behaviour in any way over this time period. It may work for Supernanny but I can assure you that it only intensified Mollie's behaviours and it was like pouring fuel on an already aggressive and out-of-control fire.

Following the battle of clothes would be the battle to get into the car. Mollie would refuse to get into the car regardless of where we were going. People would say, 'Why don't you pick her up and force her in?' The answer is that a small child kicking, pulling and hitting is very difficult to manoeuvre and restrain in a car seat. The odd time that I did manage it, she would simply unbuckle her belt and get out of the seat and hit me whilst I was driving the car.

Extreme amounts of patience were deployed in order to allow Mollie oodles of time simply to get into a car within her own timescale. Then we deployed the same amount of patience and time to allow her to make her way into her car seat in her own time. Ultimately, sitting in the car and patiently waiting while remaining silent was quicker than enduring a time-consuming and stressful full-blown meltdown. Needless to say, our days were often consumed with patiently waiting rather than actually achieving many of our objectives.

During this period we began to notice that Mollie would blatantly refuse to follow simple requests, and if she was asked not to do something she would ignore this and continue with what she was doing. She almost appeared to enjoy defying orders and would often exhibit a cheeky grin on her face when she did.

The naughty step would be the consequence for this behaviour. However, this became another battle of getting her even to stay out of the room, let alone on a step, and didn't prevent the repeat of such incidents. I really was at a complete loss with her. I would avidly watch *Supernanny* and follow all of her advice, but I was actually going backwards with Mollie rather than achieving anything. Supernanny's advice did not go down well with Mollie, and she simply became more and more challenging. Oh if only I had known then what I know now, *Supernanny* would have been banned viewing in this house!

Then Mollie, almost instantly, as if a button had been pressed, became completely obsessed with me and followed me everywhere while simultaneously demanding my constant attention. She completely cut her dad off and refused to either engage with him or to allow him to do anything for her. It goes without saying that my husband found this period extremely upsetting. She craved complete and total one-on-one attention from me, and any attempt to do anything that didn't involve her, like talking to a friend or trying to clean a room, would be repeatedly interrupted until I gave up trying either to continue or complete the task.

3

Nursery School Begins and Boom!

Mollie Aged Three to Four Years

We had hoped that with the beginning of school that Mollie's challenging behaviour would improve and the terrible twos would soon become a thing of the past. We couldn't have been more wrong!

Mollie's behaviour and our quality of life continued deteriorating during this period, and the start of school only appeared to further exacerbate an already volatile situation. Within a few months of starting nursery school, Mollie was regularly kicking teachers, staff and other children, trashing the classroom and hurling missiles across the room. It is important to note that this new and intensified level of violence began at school prior to us experiencing it at home. During her first year at mainstream nursery school Mollie was excluded approximately four times.

The school was very helpful but the staff were also at a loss with Mollie. They had not experienced anything like this before and none of the tactics successfully used on the other children had any impact on her at all. To their credit, within Mollie's first year in school the head had proactively summoned the ASD inclusion team and the educational psychologist to observe Mollie.

The educational psychologist administered the performance scale of the Wechsler Preschool and Primary Scale of Intelligence (3rd edition) and he was amazed to discover that Mollie had an IQ of 135 at 99 percentile placing her as 'very superior'. His initial conclusion was that perhaps Mollie was bored at school and needed stretching. In the years to come he would prove to be a wonderful advocate for Mollie and us.

I greatly admired his knowledge. His gentle persona put me at ease and his dedication towards the children that he encountered was clear to see. He was the first professional to say, 'I am listening and I believe you.'

Mollie's behaviour was very unpredictable. She could survive school for weeks at a time with no issues, but this period of calm would be followed by multiple incidents within the space of a week. Both the school and I were utterly and totally confused because we could not, for the life of us, understand what was causing her behaviour. There were no obvious triggers other than the fact that she appeared to need to be in complete control of her peers and she would not comply with class rules or directives.

This desire to have her needs met extended to all aspects of her life and the need for full control was gradually intensifying. Every minute of every day felt as if it was peppered with challenging behaviour, meltdowns, refusal and her constant need for control. I can remember saying to my friend as we were walking home from school. 'I can't wait for the day when I can collect Mollie from school and reach the car without a major incident occurring.'

School pickups were horrendous because she would often explode out of the school with a list of demands to be met instantly. Refusal to comply with these demands would result in a variety of actions. She might promptly attack me, kick and hit another child or just lie in the middle of the walkway leading to the main playground, screaming and refusing to move. It was also commonplace for all of the above to occur.

I would try my utmost to not respond to these behaviours, apart from her hitting other children, but simply to ignore her and walk off. Completely oblivious to her being anything other than a typically developing child with a very strong will, I would give her a consequence for her behaviour once we got home. Traditional parenting was, at that time, the only type of parenting that I knew and even though I was doing everything by the book, many assumed that I couldn't possibly be doing it correctly.

I consistently and firmly used time out, withdrawal of privileges and treats and not giving attention to negative behaviours, as well as natural consequences. Rewarding positive behaviours, giving lots of attention to desirable behaviours and using star charts were all implemented to try to reinforce positive behaviour. All failed, despite my repeated use, and using this type of behaviour modification also failed within the school setting. She just became more and more unpredictable, impulsive, defiant and out of control.

From a young age, Mollie was unbelievably jealous of others, especially if it meant that my attention was taken away from her. As a result, she would actively discourage me from having any interaction with anyone else, by means of diversion, attention-seeking behaviour, violence, damaging property and repeatedly interrupting the conversation.

During this period, Mollie was okay in public if there were plenty of things to do and few boundaries. Running around parks and play areas were still activities that she greatly enjoyed, but real difficulties in playing with peers were beginning to become more noticeable, which did make such outings increasingly stressful.

She became obsessed with her friend Gemma. Mollie would love and 'mother' Gemma, treating her as if she were her child. But, she could also instantly and without warning lash out at her, both physically and verbally. She tried to control Gemma's every move and she would also try to keep her isolated from the rest of their friendship group. Her obsession and the need for complete control over Gemma were very reminiscent of her behaviour towards me. Her behaviour towards Gemma was also causing difficulties at school because of her need to control her within the school environment. I can remember one particular meltdown at school occurring because Gemma refused to use the toilet that Mollie had told her to use. This resulted in all the children having to leave the classroom for their own safety while Mollie went around the room trashing it, like a mini tornado.

I had stopped attempting to achieve a large supermarket shop with Mollie when she was about 18 months old. It was, quite simply, a dangerous activity. When Mollie was in the supermarket trolley child seat she would continually try to get out, which concerned me in case she fell onto the hard supermarket floor.

If she was out of the supermarket trolley I couldn't shop because all of my attention and athletic agility would be spent chasing her around. She would not stay by my side and she would run around the shop laughing manically. Any attempts to encourage her to behave in an age-appropriate manner resulted in a meltdown. At 18 months old I kind of accepted this behaviour, but it was continuing as she got older and virtually all shopping had become impossible.

Simple things like family meals out were becoming more difficult to manage and were so stressful that it really wasn't worth the effort. Mollie would spend most of the evening under the table, making repeated trips to the toilet or controlling the conversation around the table, ensuring that she held centre stage. This behaviour would basically put a stop to any adult conversation. If I played with her constantly during the meal, others may have a chance to interact with each other but not to interact with me.

Mollie appeared to have no sense or idea of correct age-appropriate behaviour. We had to do normal things that other families take for granted in bite-sized chunks. We appeared to have an optimum window of time within which to achieve our 'mission', whether it was in a shop or at a doctor's appointment. Once the window of time within which acceptable behaviour was managed had been exceeded, all hell would break loose and the manic behaviour would surge to the surface.

Mollie did not play with toys as such, but preferred to act out and role play scenarios and stories. These would often be replicated scenes that she had seen on the TV, in films or in real-life scenarios, like being the teacher of a class or a dance instructor. She would always be in charge and directed family members during the role play.

She never occupied or played by herself at all and she needed constant attention. She would only play with toys or engage in other activities if she had someone to play with, usually me. When I played with Mollie, for example with dolls, she had to be in charge and would instruct me on what my doll character should say. If we were colouring in, she would instruct me on what I was allowed to colour and what colours I could use. She would also interact in this way with her peers and become aggressive and violent when they refused, tried to redirect the game or wanted any input into the theme of play.

When Mollie wanted something, she wanted it immediately and would not relent until the request had been complied with. Everything had to be instant, and not receiving this instant gratification would quickly result in an outburst of anger and frustration. When she got exited she would go into what I can only describe as 'hyper-mode' and when this happened she would become uncontrollable and completely manic.

I eventually went to the doctor's, at the school's request, to see what help was available for Mollie. The only support we could get was for my husband and I to attend a 'Triple P' parenting course. I knew that this would be a complete waste of our time and theirs. I had already attended the predecessor to Triple P several years ago when I was seeking help for my son.

I had also already tried all of the traditional parenting techniques without any long-term success, but this didn't seem to convince anyone that a Triple P course was not required. However, we did attend the course to show willing and, we hoped, to prove that whatever was going on with Mollie, it was not down to our parenting.

So a successful 38-year-old businesswoman used to dealing with staff, customers and business associates while simultaneously balancing family life with a husband with his own mental health issues (diagnosed with obsessive compulsive disorder (OCD) and later diagnosed with Asperger's), a challenging son (who was also later diagnosed with Asperger's) and challenging daughter (who would turn out to have PDA) had to endure a Triple P parenting course delivered by a very young lady with no children, who looked as if she had only just completed her university course! Impressed, I was not! Swallowing my pride and enduring the Triple P course was a hoop that I had to jump through in order to reach the next hoop. What a complete and utter waste of time and resources!

The only thing that I had in my favour to try and dispel the theory that my parenting was the root cause was the fact that the behaviour was being exhibited in two different settings – at home and at school – and that the traditional approaches used by the school and reinforced by me at home had also being unsuccessful.

It was during this time that I wrote the following passage. Without knowing it, I was already, through gut instinct, beginning to surmise where Mollie's difficulties may lie.

I have really dug my heels in with Mollie, determined to let no incident go without consequence. Because, as her parent, I know that it is my responsibility to turn this disruptive, but at the same time funny and lovable, little girl into a person who can integrate into and be accepted by society. At times Mollie's behaviour and the constant battle of wills have made me feel stressed, tense, anxious, upset and angry to the point where I have felt totally churned up and helpless inside. If Mollie's behaviour has sometimes made me feel all of the emotions above because of her constantly forcing her will against mine, is this how Mollie feels? Does she perceive the world in which she lives as constantly forcing its will against hers?

I know that this is not the case and that we are trying to teach Mollie that there are rules and correct ways to behave for her own good and well-being. However, in her little mind perhaps something is not wired correctly and in her eyes all she sees is a world full of people forcing her to do things and to behave in the ways that they want her to, taking away her control and causing the frustration to erupt into violent and aggressive meltdowns because this is the only way that she knows how to deal with these emotions.

We have tried using consequences with Mollie for her behaviour but she just doesn't seem to care. The consistent use of consequences does not modify her behaviour at all; in fact, they only seem to make things even worse.

Part 2

The School Years

4

Things Go from Bad to Worse

Mollie Aged Four to Six Years

Pre-diagnosis of Asperger's

At school, weeks of good behaviour were followed by weeks of challenging behaviour and seemed to alternate between school and home. Good behaviour at school meant that a torrent of abuse would be unleashed on me as soon as I collected her from school, and difficult behaviour at school usually meant a decrease in challenging behaviour at home. We were now realising that 'no' traditional methods of behaviour modification had any long-term effects other than to make Mollie even worse.

Mollie was again suspended on multiple occasions for violent outbursts towards staff and children and the destruction of property, because staff were concerned about the health and safety of her fellow pupils and her pregnant teacher, Mollie was removed from her class and placed in the year above. However the difficulties continued and eventually she was placed on a part-time timetable; over a period of several weeks she was only allowed to attend school for the morning period. At the suggestion of the school, I applied for a statement of special educational needs to be carried out by the local education authority (LEA). The initial request was refused, so I appealed the decision and prepared myself for a tribunal. Fortunately, several weeks before the tribunal Mollie was offered 20 hours a week of support, which was wonderful!

At home Mollie was deteriorating and regressing before my very eyes. Where had my daughter gone and who was this impostor that had taken over her body? Family tried to help, but no one could cope with the thought of looking after Mollie for more than a few hours and both of my parents worked.

As I explained to my dad, a few hours of being Mollie-free, which only occurred occasionally, was like being offered a sip of water in the middle of the Sahara – I just didn't feel the benefit of it! The noise of her screaming or shouting or the feel of her clambering all over me would often send me into a state of nervous, anxious panic.

As a family, my husband and I both felt very isolated and alone. There was no one to talk to who understood how stressful and draining life felt at that moment. Even our family didn't, at that time, understand the impact that Mollie had on our lives because they didn't live with her 24/7.

By now, Child and Adolescent Mental Health Services (CAMHS) were seeing Mollie on a regular basis. But none of the strategies that they asked us to implement had any long-term success and they were not forthcoming with any sort of assessment process or referral. In short, I felt stuck and I felt I was getting nowhere fast with CAMHS.

The CAMHS therapist I was seeing was lovely and was trying to help. I don't have any issues with his efforts, but most sessions were spent with me in tears and him counselling me, rather than either of us coming up with anything productive for Mollie. How many times can you keep repeating the words, 'I have already tried that and it doesn't work?' CAMHS could not offer me anything that I had not already done but did not suggest alternatives. I once again felt that, because no assessment or diagnosis was being offered, my parenting was the main focus.

Mollie's educational psychologist and Sue from the ASD inclusion team suggested Asperger's as a possible diagnosis. Even though I could see that she didn't quite fit the profile, I still grabbed it with both hands as a possible lifeline so that I could help my daughter.

CAMHS were still not suggesting anything new and were continually going over the same old ground; I was becoming increasingly frustrated and desperate. Looking back, I suppose that due to PDA, and even a female profile of autism spectrum disorder (ASD), being virtually unheard of back then, my CAMHS therapist was simply at a loss about how to help me. There also appeared to be a strong ethos within my local CAMHS not to diagnose or label children, which I still find rather strange. Fortunately, Mollie's wonderful educational psychologist offered to refer Mollie for an Asperger's assessment with the ASD diagnostic team.

I was on my knees by this stage and really struggling to hold myself together. Fortunately, my husband phoned our local autism support group and even though we didn't yet have a diagnosis, they welcomed us with open arms. My local Asperger's/Autism Association were, during this period, my saviours.

They helped me through an extremely difficult time and I will always be so thankful for the shoulders to cry on and the support I was offered. They referred me to social services for urgent support due to my own crumbling mental health and stated that we were 'a family in crisis'.

Unfortunately, no support was forthcoming because we had no official diagnosis. This is something else that I find baffling about CAMHS's reluctance to diagnose: without a diagnosis families cannot access the support that they may need through various outside agencies.

Life was, by now, becoming impossible and the meltdowns were growing in their frequency and intensity. I became very focused on reading and watching anything that I could about ASD in general. Mollie's educational psychologist had a particular interest in ASD and he would frequently lend me books.

I did once ask him where his interest in ASD had originated, and he told me that when he had been studying to become a psychologist, his professor and mentor had a special interest in this field, which had filtered down to himself. I would learn in the years to come that Mollie's dear and wonderful educational psychologist had been taught alongside Phil Christie by Professor Elizabeth Newson!

One evening I enthusiastically turned on the TV to watch a documentary called *Young, Autistic and Stagestruck*. Wow – right there and right then and on that very show – I first laid my eyes on the only child I had ever seen who resembled my daughter. This particular child, coincidentally also named Molly, was diagnosed with something called PDA. I eagerly googled this condition and experienced my 'light-bulb' moment. Here, for the first time, was a cluster of symptoms and behaviours that looked as if they had been specifically written for my daughter.

With no hesitation I excitedly called the ASD assessment team to tell them of my discovery but disappointingly I was informed that PDA was not recognised as being a genuine diagnosis within my local health authority and that it was a diagnosis only given in Nottingham. Because they were the professionals, who at that time I trusted and respected, I believed them and I dropped any further pursuit of PDA. Big mistake!

This decision not to investigate or consider the possibility of PDA because it was not in a diagnostic manual caused both my daughter and I another year of hell and regression by having the wrong diagnosis and the wrong strategies.

PDA was not as well represented or as well known back then, so I can understand why professionals didn't feel that they could actually assess or diagnose a child with PDA. However what I can't understand is the fact that the PDA cluster of symptoms and behaviours were not even investigated, as far as I know, as a possibility for Mollie, given the complexity of her presentation and the difficulties that I was reporting. Simply reading the diagnostic profile of PDA in conjunction with my written reports of Mollie's behaviours would surely have been enough for someone to say, 'We can't officially diagnose anything other than Asperger's but we can unofficially explore this possibility and the recommended strategies for children who present with the PDA profile due to the huge similarity between my reports of Mollie and the PDA diagnostic profile.'

Instead, the assessment for Asperger's went ahead as planned and at the age of six years old, she was officially diagnosed with Asperger's syndrome. As we were struggling to cope with our present situation, my local ASD diagnostic team referred us to social services for extra support.

I was, however, disappointed that no specific additional medical help, in the form of helping us to cope and deal with Mollie, was offered. I was offered a 'Wise Up' course, but I couldn't attend it because I was housebound with

Mollie. I also didn't know what a course could offer me with regard to Asperger's that I hadn't already read and educated myself on. My difficulty and area of need wasn't that I needed to learn about ASD, but that I needed to see someone who could investigate why, even with a lot of ASD knowledge, understanding and applied strategies, she was simply regressing, becoming more violent and spiralling out of control!

Post-diagnosis of Asperger's

At school, even with her diagnosis of Asperger's, the implementation of ASD strategies and a statement of special educational needs giving her 20 hours of support a week, things didn't improve but went steadily downhill.

Mollie was insisting that I, not her dad, took her to school; once we arrived she would find it extremely difficult to leave me and needed a teddy with her all day. She would cling onto me for dear life and was, on occasion, physically removed from my arms kicking and screaming. My heart felt as if it was breaking into a thousand pieces and I would walk home viewing the world through teary eyes.

Getting Mollie into school was proving more and more difficult and it was common for us to arrive at anytime between 11.00am and 12.00 noon. It was also common for her to kick someone on purpose so that she could return straight home. We were beginning to enter the phenomenon of 'school refusal'.

It was at this point that I decided that continually forcing Mollie into school was nothing short of mental torture for her. With the full support of the services involved, I removed Mollie from mainstream school and requested a specialised placement.

Meanwhile, at home in the months following her diagnosis, Mollie was becoming even more physically and verbally aggressive to everyone around her. We were having huge battles at bedtime and she was still awake and wreaking havoc into the early hours.

She was also regularly stealing other people's belongings and either hiding them or throwing them away. Much to my horror, she had started urinating on beds, towels and so on. Shops were now impossible, due to the huge public meltdowns that she had when I put a limit on how much money I was prepared to spend.

The control was spreading, even down to where we all sat in the car, in what order we were allowed to walk down the street and which direction we should take when we were out and about.

It was during this period that Blueberry Bear was born. Blueberry was a blue cuddly bear, who became a very real persona in her own right. She was initially used by Mollie as an enticement to encourage other children to play with her, but she quickly became her constant companion and her only friend.

During this period, Mollie also began to 'skin pick', which, I have read, is associated with high anxiety. Her face and arms became covered in scabs, some of which have left scars.

As a family, we found ourselves constantly trying to go with the flow while simultaneously making all sorts of accommodations and concessions for her, simply to try to prevent a meltdown. We were beaten, drained and exhausted. I could not find any evidence of this type of complex and extreme behaviour regarding this level of control, and the subsequent backlash if it was is not forthcoming, in my considerable research on Asperger's.

When Mollie was three I had my first taste of not being able to cope. I would pick myself up and start again, trying to think of new strategies to deal and cope with her behaviour. These episodes of hopelessness, extreme anxiety and desperation were now occurring on a more regular basis with shorter gaps in between. My optimism that I would eventually come across a method that would help me manage Mollie's behaviour successfully was all but gone. My fuse was shorter, and I would snap and shout more regularly. I felt trapped by her behaviour and physically and mentally exhausted. Following my dad's retirement and with the true extent of Mollie's difficulties fully recognised, I received excellent help and support from all of my family, without whom I would have gone under.

I became convinced that if Mollie did, as I had been told, have Asperger's then it couldn't possibly be 'travelling alone'. On several occasions I queried with my local ASD diagnostic team the fact that Mollie appeared to be regressing and I questioned whether she could have attention deficit hyperactivity disorder (ADHD), as well as Asperger's, because of the complexity of her presentation. She was relentlessly on the go and constantly fidgeting. I was unable to engage her attention on one activity for long; we constantly had to chop and change what we were doing in order to keep her focused. If she was watching the TV, the minute the adverts came on she required constant attention from me because she couldn't cope with the boredom of a three-minute advert break.

My enquiry about ADHD, and the suggestion that parents should perhaps be offered the opportunity to have this investigated if they were reporting extreme and challenging behaviour, was about as well received as my query regarding PDA. I was informed that any evidence of

ADHD would have been noticed and highlighted during an individual's previous assessments and observations.

Following complaints from Mollie that certain colours hurt her eyes and concern expressed by my mum that Mollie appeared to be memorising rather than reading books I arranged for Mollie to have an eye test performed by an 'orthoscopic optician'. This eye test confirmed that Mollie had major visual perception difficulties, which basically meant that she had features consistent with Irlen syndrome and dyslexia.

She was prescribed a pair of glasses with a red lens that calmed the over-stimulation and visual disturbances that she was experiencing. I began to investigate other possible sensory issues in case these were also adding to her distress at school. Why, oh why, did nobody think to inform me during her assessment for Asperger's about the likelihood of accompanying sensory issues? Why was I discovering this several months on through my own investigations? Surely it makes common sense when any individual is diagnosed with any ASD for the clinicians involved to inform parents about the possibility of sensory issues and maybe even supply them with some accompanying literature! However, to be fair, when I mentioned these sensory issues to the ASD diagnostic team, they did refer her to an occupational therapist for further investigation.

Disillusioned, and a little bit in shock at the apparent apathy towards my plight from the ASD diagnostic team, I consulted Mollie's educational psychologist and asked his opinion regarding my concerns. I explained to him that Mollie's behaviour was still deteriorating and I suggested the possibility that she may have a co-morbid disorder that was perpetuating the problem.

He cautiously suggested PDA, perhaps under the assumption that I had never heard of it. I was amazed and relieved that he, without me mentioning it to him, could also see the traits. I explained that my local ASD team had basically told me that it wasn't a real condition and that it was only diagnosed in Nottingham, to which he replied, 'Oh it is a real condition, a very real one indeed.' It was only at this point that I learned about his previous connections to Phil Christie and Professor Elizabeth Newson. He also made the point that PDA was not a co-morbid condition, as such, but was simply a different subgroup/condition within the 'family of pervasive developmental disorders' and that Mollie wouldn't necessarily have Asperger's and PDA but that she may simply have PDA.

Following this seal of approval, I forwarded the Elizabeth Newson Centre an email with Mollie's developmental profile. Phil Christie replied that these behaviours were consistent with PDA and that a referral seemed appropriate and would contribute to a better understanding of Mollie's profile and needs.

For some reason – I really don't know why – I put this on the back-burner and did not revisit it or actively pursue an assessment of PDA until some six months later. We were in the process of moving house and both my husband and son were experiencing debilitating mental health issues at the time. I guess that there was just so much going on that keeping my head above water was all I could manage to do. However, I began to use the strategies for supporting children with PDA originally proposed by Elizabeth Newson and subsequently developed by colleagues at the centre. These strategies advocate a less directive and more flexible approach than is usually suggested for children with a more typical presentation of autism.

Maybe the failings of CAMHS and the ASD diagnostic team, in my case, to offer me anything in the way of services to actually help and understand my daughter were down to a combination of difficulties. At that time, there was not the amount of information available on PDA as there is now, limited funding can perhaps make it difficult to provide individuals with a more personalised approach rather than a set pathway and professionals do appear to have to follow a directive of following a set approach/ pathway imposed on them from a higher power.

Whatever the reason or wherever the directives originated from, I felt like a product on a conveyor belt in a production line. There appeared to be no personal touch or individual approach. I felt as if I was simply being churned through a set and rigid process that had no flexibility or adaptability for the individual or anything that didn't neatly fit in a set box.

5

A New School and a New Start

Mollie Aged Seven to Eight Years

Pre-diagnosis of PDA

Mollie was at home full time for a period of 15 months while a new school was sourced and prepared and a very gradual introduction to the staff and the school took place. At home I had begun using PDA strategies but, looking back, I feel that she was in such a dark place that the use of choice and options just wasn't enough to reach her and grab her out of the black hole that was sucking her in. In the future, I would learn more about PDA and realise that Mollie needed more individualised support and strategies than the generic PDA ones. I am sure that this is something that many parents will identify with.

It was during this period that Mollie's fantasy life and role play reached a whole new intensity. Blueberry Bear was real and we had to treat her, at all times, like Mollie's baby sister. Lies and tales of fantasy were now becoming more elaborate and more a part of normal everyday functioning. Any activity that we attempted to do with Mollie was transformed to a role play scenario written, produced and directed by Mollie. When she was in new situations Mollie's behaviour would regresses to that of a much younger child – sitting on my knee, talking in a baby voice and so on.

We had recently moved house and a neighbour's child had been coming round to play, which had proved to be disastrous. Mollie completely controlled this child and lashed out at her on a regular basis. When I intervened, to protect the other child, Mollie would often go into a complete meltdown and the level of violence, intensity and duration of each meltdown was indescribable. She had become obsessed with this child and every waking minute of Mollie's life was spent waiting for her to arrive at our house.

When Mollie found herself in new situations with children who she did not know, she could be very verbally and physically aggressive with them, especially if they were attempting to engage her. Looking back, I suppose that the other child initiating the interaction was, in itself, seen as a demand by Mollie.

Mollie hated unexpected visitors at the house and other people speaking to me, in case they were trying to steal me from her. She would resort to various tactics to get them to leave – bombarding conversations with interruptions, questions and noise, spraying water on them, removing her clothes, using rude language, telling them to get out and physical violence.

Mollie was 'only' manageable if interaction with her was one on one and her needs were being met, that is, she was in control. The house had become a fortress designed to keep us both socially isolated and, therefore, to keep anxieties low. Communication between Jake, Lee and I was constantly interrupted and bombarded by attention-seeking behaviour, as were my phone calls.

The phone was usually answered by Mollie, who would then inform the caller that she was 'home alone'. On the odd occasion that I did reach the phone before her, she would promptly pull the plug out of the wall. Her mood would change rapidly from happy to aggressive as soon as a new need was not met or when the smallest of demands was made of her. Mollie used behaviour and avoidance to express her emotions and anxieties rather than speech. Everything in Mollie's day-to-day living had to be negotiated, and goalposts were repeatedly moved. Mollie was at her most contented at home with one-on-one company and no longer wanted to go to parks or play areas.

Mollie was happy and content if the day's events were completely on her terms and were facilitated within her timescale. This made normal, day-to-day living impossible, which, of course, resulted in outbursts. Mollie did not appear to have any concern for the feelings or emotions of other people, and the world truly revolved around her. Even though I had reduced the anxiety caused by sensory issues, mainstream school and unnecessary changes in routine, and I was providing activities that didn't require social interaction (unless Mollie chose it) and using PDA strategies, Mollie's outbursts and difficulties continued to escalate.

Mollie's usual way of communicating with me was by screaming and shouting. Even simple questions like, 'Is your film good?' would be answered with, 'Get out you git!' On most days we were having two or three meltdowns that involved screaming, shouting, trashing and damaging property, hitting, kicking and throwing objects at me. These objects could be phones, remote controls and even knives, cups and plates.

The rest of the day would be spent trying to avoid, defuse or de-escalate any further outbursts. Meltdowns were long-drawn-out episodes, often lasting for hours rather than minutes. The worst meltdown that I ever experienced lasted for five hours, exhausting for both of us. Going out became virtually impossible because Mollie refused to leave the house. During this period, Mollie reluctantly agreed to take melatonin to help with her increasing sleep problems.

She was also beginning to struggle more with activities outside of the home. For about a year, my dad and I had both been taking Mollie to a 'special needs playground' every Saturday afternoon to ensure that she was having adequate social interaction. This started to cause problems, with multiple meltdowns while she was there, which eventually resulted in her deciding not to go anymore.

Mollie was also attending a special needs club every Wednesday evening. It was based at the special needs playground and had a soft play area, outdoor playground and arts and crafts. Because this was a club, there were fewer visitors than there would be at the playground on a Saturday afternoon. However, within a few months she was having meltdowns here, which, for the safety of others, resulted in her being locked in the soft play area while they waited for me to collect her. Needless to say, she never went back.

When Mollie was seven I officially gave up work, following a year of very intermittent attendance, and concentrated all of my time and attention solely on Mollie. I officially became Mollie's full-time carer and because she refused to leave the home, I was, for all intents and purposes, completely housebound.

My mum and dad have given, and continue to give, me the most amazing support and unfortunately their lives were also dramatically affected by Mollie's behaviour. They were both in their sixties and instead of enjoying retirement, they were doing as much as they could to help me. They would not even book a holiday because they knew how fragile my own mental health was.

When I told the ASD diagnostic team that Mollie was still not improving and had commented that she became stressed with her friend because she didn't understand Mollie's words, they carried out a speech and language comprehension assessment for her, which came back as average, so there were no concerns there.

Following the referral to social services as a 'family in crisis', due to my rapidly deteriorating mental health, we were finally awarded two hours a week of respite, delivered by their outreach services. Mollie's outreach workers were to become the most wonderful advocates for Mollie, PDA and our family as a whole. They fought my corner and supported me every step of the way, and I will always be very grateful.

I had already conducted a lot of research into sensory issues and read several books, so I was not surprised when the occupational therapist found that Mollie exhibited many of the behaviours that are consistent with difficulties across multiple senses and she was diagnosed with sensory processing disorder.

It was at this point that I decided to revisit PDA and seek a diagnostic assessment. My faith in my local services, further exacerbated by difficulties that I was now experiencing with Jake, was now non-existent. This had not been helped by the fact that the more I learned, the more I realised how little the professionals actually appeared to know.

Prior to appealing for funding for an out-of-area assessment at the Elizabeth Newson Centre, my local services arranged to meet to discuss Mollie and PDA. Given my lack of faith in the local services, and the fact that only a year ago they had said that PDA didn't exist, I didn't want to risk them deciding to do the assessment themselves so I asked my GP to refer Mollie for a private assessment at the Elizabeth Newson Centre.

I joined the PDA Society Forum (previously the PDA Contact Group Forum) so that I could try to learn and understand more from other parents. It is worth noting that, even though I had stated that I no longer required any involvement from my local ASD team, they still continued to attend Mollie's review meetings with my permission.

By December of that year, I had raised the prospect of PDA with Mollie's proposed new school and had explained that I was going to seek a diagnosis for PDA. At that point, Mollie was not yet attending this school because of the preparation and funding that needed to be put into place for her. However, I informed the staff so that they could begin to learn about PDA and the prospect that using PDA strategies may be the most successful approach for Mollie.

In January of the following year, the new school had allocated Mollie her special needs teacher, who began to do home visits with Mollie to establish a relationship. Within a couple of months she had introduced Mollie to the lady who would be her teaching assistant (TA), and these visits continued at home until the school felt that both they and Mollie were ready to start visits to the actual school.

Mollie's educational psychologist continued to review and observe Mollie at home and just before her assessment at the Elizabeth Newson Centre, he conducted a full-scale Wechsler Intelligence Scale Test For Children (4th edition), which concluded that Mollie had a full-scale IQ of 123 at 94 percentile.

Post-diagnosis of PDA

In May, at the age of seven years and seven months, Mollie was diagnosed with PDA by Phil Christie and his team at the Elizabeth Newson Centre. To say that I felt truly vindicated would be an understatement, but the most important aspect for me was that I now had a diagnosis that accurately described my daughter and her difficulties and signposted others to the correct understanding and strategies.

The assessment process at the Elizabeth Newson Centre was a lovely experience. At last I felt that I was in the hands of professionals who actually knew what they were doing. They quite clearly had a much deeper understanding of ASD than the surface-level knowledge that I had previously encountered with other diagnostic clinicians. I actually felt warmth, compassion and understanding from Phil Christie and his team during this assessment, towards both myself and Mollie.

Before the day of the assessment, staff had contacted me to get as much information as they could about Mollie so that they could prepare for the assessment and put us all at ease. They also contacted the other professionals who had been involved to get copies of reports and their views. On the day of the assessment, Mollie was in the playroom with one of the psychologists for around four hours, with a short break. We were able to see all that was happening through the one-way screen, while we were asked questions about Mollie's history and how she was at home. Another member of the team took detailed notes of everything Mollie did and the report that we received included an analysis of this, as well as the discussion that we had. This meant we could clearly see how and why the diagnosis was made.

As soon as Mollie was diagnosed with PDA, the ASD diagnostic team immediately discharged Mollie from their services and told me to seek any further help for Mollie from alternative agencies. We had effectively been dumped! That was fine by me, but I thought that it was strange because they had continued with their involvement up until this point. I called to ask why this had been done and was informed that it was because they didn't feel that they could offer any advice for a child with PDA, because I had said that typical ASD strategies did not work for her. I offered to draw a line under our past experiences and to move on from them. I also offered them full access to Mollie if they wished to learn more about PDA and to effectively use her for the purpose of research in the hope that this may help other children. I never heard anything back, so this wonderful opportunity, that could have benefitted those who may follow in her footsteps, was wasted.

Eventually, towards the end of July, Mollie's new school had everything in place for her and we could start introducing her to the school. Mollie and I made visits to the school consisting of just two hours a week. I initially stayed on the premises, until Mollie was happy for me to leave her. We gradually built these up from two hours to three hours a week, a morning a week and then a full day a week. Then we progressed from one day a week to two days a week and so on. Before we knew it the summer holidays had arrived and it was time for a break until the new school year began.

Through the PDA Society (previously the PDA Contact Group) and in particular a fellow parent, Neville Starnes, I was able to build up a gradual and steady understanding of Mollie and why she behaved the way that she did. I needed more than the diagnostic profile and generic strategies; I needed a full-blown understanding and to develop those generic strategies into a unique programme for Mollie. Unfortunately, I was powerless to halt PDA's rapid and damaging progression, due to the external stimuli that lay outside our window.

At home, Mollie had become obsessed with the street and the children in it. She could not cope with playing with them but could not cope without them. She would control to an extreme level, tell tales of fantasy that the older ones did not believe, resort to kicking and hitting, verbally and physically attacking me when I tried to intervene, tell me to shut my face in front of other parents, throw buckets of water over me, attacking me in public and reduce toddlers to tears, and that is just the tip of the iceberg.

I knew that I must be the main focal point of gossip in my street and understandably so. Most of my neighbours were very nice and supportive and have continued to be this way. However, this did nothing to lessen my embarrassment and the sense of shame that I felt for not being able to control my own child.

Things got worse and worse. Children were now actively trying to get rid of her when she went out to play. Other children soon learnt which buttons to press in order to prompt a reaction from Mollie. I can understand why they wanted to exclude her from their play, but it was heartbreaking all the same.

The other tragedy was that she was being vilified for behaviours that were actually being carefully instigated by others. As this continued, so the intensities of the meltdowns increased even further. She would fly in, trash the house, use me as a punch bag, scream obscenities into my face and demand I go out and chastise other people's children or tell off their parents. This would go on for hour after hour. A full vocabulary of swear-words was now beginning to emerge and she would use them at will with no regard to age or authority.

It is only as I look back and write this that I can honestly say that I truly do not know how either Lee or I continued to go on day after day while still trying to provide a life for Jake. He also bore witness to all of this, as did his friends, which is why we so vehemently tried to protect his personal life from Mollie's influence.

My parents were by now daily visitors to my house, offering much-needed breaks and respite. Without them I simply would not have coped and how those without parental support cope, I simply do not know.

It was awful – my most private of difficulties played out in a grand performance before an audience of neighbours in a street that I had only recently moved into. My own mental health reached its lowest point and I could neither physically nor mentally cope with Mollie any longer. Hell, I couldn't cope with anything any longer, and I knew that I was on the verge of cracking. I was having suicidal thoughts and I was fearful of hurting Mollie, because the urge to strike back when she was attacking me was becoming harder and harder to suppress.

My parents took Mollie to stay with them for a few days to offer her some love and reassurance while simultaneously giving Lee and I a break. We had rapidly reached the point of no return and simply could not go on any longer.

Social services arranged for Mollie to be placed in emergency respite for a week. We sold this to her as a break for her away from the street so that she could enjoy some calm days. She went happily and we visited her every day while she was there. She knew that we would pick her up if things got too much for her to cope with.

It was during these darkest of times that Lee and I both wept and faced the awful possibility that our only option, due to our complete inability to cope anymore, may be to place Mollie in care. All I could see was a lifetime ahead of me being abused and hit by my own daughter and I just couldn't cope with her anymore.

Mollie came home from emergency respite and we continued trying to claw our way from one day to another. We were barely existing, let alone living. Due to the seriousness of our situation social services agreed to fund overnight respite for Mollie one weekend a month. So we accessed a monthly weekend respite break but Mollie refused to go back. As a result of Mollie refusing the weekend respite, I requested that the funding that we weren't using for overnight respite should instead be given to us in the form of direct payments. I was initially awarded three hours a week support via direct payments but this was increased to seven hours within a few months. She continued to play in the street and the meltdowns continued on a daily basis.

In October, Mollie, at last, began attending her second school. We experienced a very promising start but the telltale signs that all was not well began to slowly emerge after a few months.

She had a statement of special educational needs giving her 50 hours of support. This provided her with full-time support throughout the whole school day for five days a week with two full-time teaching assistants. She was also provided with her own room to spend time in, and she could chose whether she wanted to go into class or stay in her room and choose an activity there. I must point out that my LEA did everything that they could to adequately support Mollie in school – they readily supplied the funding, her educational psychologist became more like a family friend who supported and advocated for us every step of the way and her new school and teachers were nothing short of tremendous.

At school, Mollie was always dealt with in a calm and loving manner, even following a meltdown, and was made to feel that she was a very valued member of the school by all of the staff. Great care was taken to help Mollie develop positive peer relationships. She accessed classroom learning whenever she chose to do so or had positive interactions and learning with her TAs in her own room.

Every day would present Mollie and her TAs with new challenges, which we would work on together as a team. Mollie still had difficult days that would result in very challenging behaviour, both verbally and physically. However, she was no longer suspended or sent home but was instead helped to move on and learn from such incidents.

I could now have a break in the daytime but I just couldn't seem to rebuild my strength, and within a very short period the respite of school was being erased by increasing struggles at home. Getting her to school was proving to be a nightmare, with more avoidance and anxiety-prompting outbursts each morning.

There were frequent phone calls in the day demanding this, that and the other from Mollie, so I could sometimes be trotting to and from the school up to three times a day. She would often phone me up demanding to be collected from school, and if I didn't pick her up the carnage when I did arrive was unbelievable.

There would be a trashed room, graffiti and vulgar language written on her windows and teachers banned from the room having both been physically and verbally attacked. One of her TAs could only cope for a few months before needing to be reallocated to a different child.

Picking Mollie up from school was nothing short of a nightmare due to suppressed anxiety and difficulties transitioning from the school to the car. This would cause blowouts in the street or being locked out of my car followed by demands for toys to be purchased before she would agree to come home. The school pickup could take me between two and three hours, and it was only a 15-minute drive away.

She had become fixated on a child in her class and the same pattern of behaviour was repeating itself. She was obsessed with this girl, needed to control her and was trying to isolate her from the group. When the other child didn't respond and began to withdraw from Mollie, this crushed her self-esteem, so she would react by lashing out at this child.

Her other original TA eventually required a week off work due to stress, such were the tremendous emotional difficulties associated with managing Mollie on a daily basis. The new headmistress was deeply concerned about the effect that Mollie was having on her staff and the other children and tentatively suggested that perhaps Mollie's needs would be better met in a specialised provision. She was lovely and very caring in her approach to me; she simply had the best interests of all concerned at heart.

The school continued to experience more incidents and eventually staff were forced to restrain her to stop her from attacking a member of staff and from trying to run off. When I arrived she was having a full panic attack and was like a cornered, frightened animal. In hindsight, all Mollie wanted to do was to find a safe place to be alone; she wasn't running off, she was simply seeking sanctuary. The staff chased her because they were afraid for her safety, which, of course, intensified Mollie's anxiety, resulting in her attacking one of the staff chasing her.

Mollie refused to go back because of her fear of restraint and the humiliation that the incident had caused her. Mollie commented to me, 'I don't fit in here anymore, I don't fit in anywhere. I need a school where other kids are like me.'

So in May, this wonderful school placement, that could not have possibly done anything more for her, ended in school refusal. Despite the use of everything recommended for a successful placement for a child with PDA, it was still too much for Mollie to cope with. We went back to home visits from her TAs to try and re-establish and repair relationships, but she eventually refused these also.

It was during this time that Mollie stopped playing in the street, which was a huge relief to me as this had become the source of most of the meltdowns that we encountered at home.

During Mollie's time at her second school placement, recognising the early warning signs that she was struggling to cope, I had consulted Mollie's paediatrician to discuss possible medication and to once again consider whether she may also have ADHD as a co-morbid condition.

The paediatrician was hopeful that medication may help Mollie and a referral was made back to CAMHS with a view to assess for ADHD and to medicate. In March, we'd had our appointment with CAMHS and they agreed to refer Mollie to the local psychiatry services.

Several months later we attended an appointment with the psychiatry service, fully expecting Mollie to begin an assessment for ADHD with a view to medicating, depending on the results of that assessment.

The psychiatrist informed me that he was well informed about me and my past dealings with Connect (one of the three services that parents can access with children who are appearing to struggle with mental health issues), CAMHS and the ASD diagnostic team. He refused point-blank to discuss Mollie, saying that this was due to his lack of experience with PDA. He suggested that Mollie be referred to an out-of-area hospital where they did have experience of PDA. He continued to explain that a request for funding would need to go to a panel and that I may need to pay for the appointment myself!

To add further insult to injury, he went on to say that the local health authority would not be prepared to monitor any medication that may be prescribed by the hospital that he was recommending he refer Mollie to. This would mean frequent trips to and from this out-of-area hospital for the straightforward monitoring of any potential medication.

It took every ounce of resilience that I could summon not to fall apart during that appointment and to remain calm and dignified. I had patiently waited for six months from my first enquiry about medication and an ADHD assessment just to be told that nothing was going to be done locally and to be subjected to a dismissive approach from the psychiatrist. I left the appointment in a state of shock and I broke down in tears as soon as I reached the safety of our car.

I may be wrong, but the actions of that day left me with the feeling that, perhaps due to previous disputes with my local health services, I had been completely blackballed. Unfortunately, the only victim in all of this was an eight-year-old child.

6

An End to Formal Education

Mollie Aged Eight to Ten Years

After the breakdown of Mollie's second school placement, I was in bits and just couldn't carry on with Mollie at home any longer. We sought a residential placement for Mollie in the hope that she would be better looked after and supported by a team of people, rather than by one shattered, destroyed and short-tempered mum. I knew that I was not giving her what she needed and that we were spiralling into a black hole of mutual resentment and extreme depression together.

The thought of going through anymore stress and anxiety was just too much for me to contemplate. I needed to have regular breaks from Mollie and, even then, the thought of going back into house arrest with a child who demanded constant attention at a manic level and who would regularly, out of nowhere, shout abuse and blow her fuse at me was just too much for me to cope with mentally.

Mollie's paediatrician bought to my attention a specialist school, which had the most fantastic facilities and, according to its website, catered for children with

PDA. The LEA agreed funding for Mollie to attend on a day placement and, following a hard-fought battle, we managed to get the funding from social services for a residential placement Monday to Friday, with Mollie returning home at the weekends and holidays. It was agreed by all parties that Mollie would, for now, attend as a day pupil only and would access the residential placement in her own time and at her own pace.

The only thing that kept me going was the thought that I would soon have some sort of life, instead of, what I can only describe as, a most terrible existence with a child who I loved but really didn't like. I was battered, bruised and crushed, and I really had nothing left to give.

Now that she was neither at school nor playing in the street, it was the first chance for us to really try and keep Mollie calm within the home. The use of PDA strategies and the exclusion of the negative external stimuli finally began to pay dividends for us and the huge meltdowns began to become a thing of the past.

When she did start her new third school in October it came as a huge relief, and the respite that school attendance offered was gratefully received. My days of rest were long because of the distance between home and school: she left the house at 8.00am and didn't return until 4.00pm. Gradually I began to replenish my depleted stores of energy and mental stability.

As expected, we had the now familiar 'honeymoon period' where, apart from an odd blip, things appeared to be going very well. We had various issues regarding the transport provided by the school, which we eventually solved with a female escort and her own taxi.

When the problems with school refusal began to resurface, it was no surprise to us. We had fully expected it due to the telltale signs that we had been noticing at home.

I now knew that if she couldn't cope at school in the day, we would have no chance of her willingly sleeping there as well.

Mollie began to struggle more and more with the expectations and perceived demands placed on her at school. She was arguing and struggling with peers, which did eventually result in her being bullied. Don't get me wrong, she can give as good as she gets, but then she can't understand why other children remain angry with her or why her behaviour then evokes a bullying mentality in others.

Before long, she was really struggling to cope with her school environment and she was finding it impossible to keep in her explosive and impulsive outbursts. She would increasingly want me to pick her up rather than come home in the taxi, which would lead to more difficulties. On one occasion we did have to collect her because the school staff just couldn't get her into the taxi, regardless of everything that they tried.

I had hoped that Mollie would enjoy the school and opportunities so much that the prospect of sleeping over and accessing all of the extra curricula activities would have made the residency desirable but this was not to be the case.

With careful handling, violent meltdowns were a thing of the past at home, but the explosive verbal outbursts and extreme control continued. Difficult days at school only exacerbated what was already challenging behaviour. The school refusal started again and the extreme anxiety that she was enduring by just trying to go into school was very evident.

The residential placement never even got off the ground, and by then I had realised that this was not the correct placement for Mollie. The only placement that Mollie could cope with was 'Home'.

One thing led to another and eventually she was just unable to continue attending school, because her anxieties and inability to control her own reactions had, once again, led to complete school refusal.

I was asked by the other services involved to chase up Mollie's out-of-area appointment with a view to medication. It became apparent that the promise to refer out of area and to apply for funding had never been processed or followed up. Following several phone calls requesting that Mollie now be assessed for ADHD locally and that any medication prescribed by the out-of-area hospital should be monitored locally, while simultaneously accusing my local services of gross neglect in their duty of care, I finally started to see some progress. The out-of-area hospital was finally officially approached to assess and discuss Mollie with a view to medication. My local services agreed to assess for possible co-morbid ADHD and to monitor any medication that the out-of-area hospital may prescribe.

It was now 15 months since I had first requested medication from Mollie's paediatrician and ten months since my disastrous appointment with the psychiatrist and his promise to refer her to an out-of-area hospital!

Fortunately, Mollie's short burst of school attendance had allowed my depleted batteries to be recharged enough for me to make the very big decision to keep her at home and to give up on any further school placements. I wrote to the LEA requesting that her name be removed from the school register.

This is when we saw a big change in Mollie. With the prospect of never having to attend a school again, we entered our calmest waters. I could now cope with Mollie because she was calmer and less explosive than she had ever been before.

Since the purchase of an iPad and developing a fascination with Netflix, Mollie had become far less demanding of everybody's attention and the constant need to be entertained had diminished. She would occupy herself by watching back-to-back TV show episodes on her iPad while simultaneously colouring in or building Lego. When she interacted with me, the iPad would often be on in the background otherwise she would appear to struggle to concentrate and flit from one thing to another.

She still refused to leave the house and appeared to need this fake environment – of home – to stabilise her internal system. She could still be impulsive but this was more evident in her verbal outbursts than anything else. By excluding the external stimulation of the outside world, her general system had become more stable and calm.

However, remove her from this bubble and place her back in a normal environment, and the problems with boredom, control, anxiety, impulsiveness and manic behaviour would return. We continued to see spikes in controlling, hyperactive and impulsive behaviours if we had an event approaching that she was looking forward to. The weeks leading up to Christmas, Easter, holidays and so on would always see a return of these behaviours.

But we weren't out of stormy waters yet, and the following year would be a rollercoaster of emotions, self-discovery, depression and acute social anxiety!

Part 3

Understanding Mollie's PDA Behaviours

7

Difficulties with Social Understanding and Verbal Communication

By the age of ten Mollie was doing much better and our lives had finally become liveable. There was still plenty of learning, nurturing and work to be done, but the steps forward that we had made were massive.

One of the biggest steps forward, for me, was to really try to understand and see the world through Mollie's eyes so that I could understand her behaviour. I could see the results of her difficulties by her need to control and avoid, her impulsiveness and her meltdowns but I couldn't understand why daily living would evoke such a strong reaction to the point where everything and anything had to be either avoided at all costs or on her terms only.

I am not a qualified professional, and my opinions are solely based on the experiences of living with a child with PDA and the shared experiences of other parents. Therefore some of these interpretations may be unique to Mollie but may apply to other children with PDA as well.

So let's look at some of the difficulties that seem to underpin Mollie's profile of PDA and the subsequent behaviours that she shows. Why don't we all try and put ourselves in Mollie's shoes? After all, aren't we the ones with supposedly superior empathy?

Difficulty with social understanding and interacting

One of the differences that set children with PDA apart from other children with a more typical presentation of ASD is that they appear to have better social understanding and empathy. They can use this understanding and empathy to predict how someone else may react in order to avoid demands or to manipulate situations. However, this can appear to be at an intellectual level rather than an emotional one.

Indeed, the pattern of social insight and social difficulty presents a real clinical puzzle. On the one hand, Machiavellian manipulation implies good social insight. Yet these children also display a striking absence of embarrassment, lack a sense of the need to conform socially and show difficulties judging their place in the social hierarchy. This could imply that, while most children with ASD show deficits in 'theory of mind', those with PDA have problems selectively impairing other aspects of socio-cognitive processing (O'Nions 2014).

Mollie appears to have an abundance of empathy and social understanding when it comes to using it for her own purposes but genuinely appears to have great difficulty in actually feeling things from another person's perspective. Other than appearing to have good social insight in order to manipulate, avoid and control, which may be learned at an intellectual level, Mollie does appear to have very real difficulties with other areas of social understanding, which causes her huge difficulties with social interaction.

Mollie is naturally a very sociable child, who wants to be able to interact, have friends and go to play areas and parties. But there is a snag: although she wants to do these things, she just doesn't appear to understand intuitively how to do them. While certain areas of her social insight are strong, other areas appear to be very weak, which means that, for Mollie, social empathy and understanding is somewhat of a paradox.

Mollie does appear to have a complete lack of self-identity and sense of who she is combined with not intuitively knowing how to behave, which must be a cause of her huge anxiety and confusion. If the natural Mollie has no sense of embarrassment, social compulsion or social hierarchy then she may appear very confusing and rude to others but at the same time completely normal to herself.

The sorts of behaviour that these difficulties elicit are not going to win Mollie friends any time soon and did result in Mollie repeatedly being told off. When Mollie is simply being herself in social situations everything appears to go wrong for her but she may not intuitively know why.

Speaking out of turn, interrupting, controlling, invading someone's personal space, snatching things off people, having no respect for adults, treating her peers as if she is the adult, insisting that rules are followed by others but then blatantly ignoring them herself and being very overfamiliar with people in an inappropriate manner, for example sitting on the knee of an adult who she doesn't know very well or one in a position of authority, are all behaviours that others may find rude, puzzling and unacceptable.

How confusing it must be for Mollie when these behaviours are what come naturally and instinctively to her. This is who she is, and she doesn't know any different. How awful it must be for Mollie to be consistently reprimanded and punished for simply being who she is naturally programmed to be. Even more confusing for her may be the possibility that she has no idea why other people do not deem her behaviours as acceptable because she can't intuitively understand how these behaviours are viewed or felt by others.

Is it as a result of the above difficulties that she appears to copy, mimic and imitate other children, adults or characters from TV? Is she trying to mask her huge difficulties within this area and avoid getting things wrong by copying the behaviour and characteristics of others?

Imagine Mollie's internal confusion when she is taking on the persona of a parent or teacher without understanding why this persona is not the correct one for her. Mollie may be copying the characteristics of someone who everyone else appears to find acceptable, yet when she behaves this way she is still told off, viewed as rude and deemed odd by her peers.

This effort of role playing must be exhausting. Just imagine trying to be someone that you aren't in order to fit in and not understanding why you have to do this, not to mention the possibility of still getting it wrong by inadvertently choosing the wrong persona.

When Mollie inadvertently role plays an acceptable persona, she may appear quite typical in her presentation but there may still be that little something about her that appears a little bit odd or slightly different to a neurotypical child. This is especially evident as she grows older. However, this role play can usually only be sustained for a honeymoon period, following which she finds it difficult to keep the natural her suppressed.

Does Mollie need to control the whole complex and unpredictable scenario of socialising to ensure that she doesn't do anything wrong? Is the need to know what is coming next and not to be caught out by any unexpected surprises, requests or demands one of the reasons why Mollie needs to control the actions of peers and family in order to feel secure?

Individuals playing with Mollie may simply feel as if they are actors in a play and that she is their director. She will dictate who can play with what, who can say what and, while she may give other individuals different roles to play, she always provides them with a script to follow. Is the need to control simply a mechanism to keep anxieties low in an unpredictable world or is it just a natural and intuitive part of her internal makeup?

Although when Mollie was younger she appeared to show no signs of embarrassment, the same cannot be said now. However, it is important to note that this self-awareness has developed later than you would expect in a typical child.

Mollie often appears to be deeply embarrassed over normal day-to-day interaction and speech, rather than things that a child would typically be embarrassed about. She appears to be embarrassed when her deficits in social interaction are exposed and fearful of the reactions that she may then have, which will undoubtedly draw even more attention to her.

However she still appears to not be embarrassed by things that a typically developing child may be embarrassed about. She can still display shocking behaviour like arguing with an adult in public, but she isn't embarrassed by this as long as she has control over that behaviour. She does however now feel embarrassed when she can't control her responses to events outside of her control, for example, having a meltdown or feeling humiliated if she is chastised in public and doesn't understand what she has done to elicit this reaction.

Observations and further questions

Are excessive role play, adopting a different persona, avoiding demands and controlling interactions all intrinsically linked mechanisms employed by Mollie to try and ensure that social interaction becomes predictable and therefore runs as smoothly as possible, with low anxiety and no embarrassment? Is a mix of survival, protection, anxiety, not intuitively understanding social interaction and knowing how another person may feel at an emotional level the root cause for this complex behaviour?

Alternatively, there may be an aspect of Mollie that actually does empathise at an emotional level and is aware of how her actions make others feel. After all, it is this very skill that allows her to manipulate other people in order to have her demands met or to avoid the demands of others. Perhaps the anxiety produced by not being in control overrides her ability to put the needs of anyone else before her own.

Or maybe there are aspects of both these explanations – a mixture of Mollie having empathy that is not fully developed combined with an intrinsic need to have her own needs met at the cost of all others in order to reduce anxiety levels.

I know that I have often had to role play scenarios with Mollie when she has upset me so that she can try to grasp just why I am upset or frustrated with her. When we role play the scenario and she is playing the part of me, she can be very surprised at how her behaviour feels when she is on the receiving end of it.

On one occasion she even commented, 'There is no way that I am that self-obsessed'. We were role playing how it feels for me to be shouted at every five minutes, regardless of what I am doing, to fetch and carry for her. She truly did not perceive how she was coming across to me or how it feels for the other person at an emotional level. She did, however, recognise the behaviour as being self-obsessed when she was seeing it in another person and it was being directed at her.

Misinterpreting verbal communication

Children with PDA can appear more fluent with language and have better social timing than you would expect to see in children with a typical presentation of ASD. However, children with PDA still appear to have difficulties within this area of communication.

While the majority of children with PDA develop very fluent expressive language, some do not have such robust understanding. It is not so much that they do not understand the language that is used (i.e. that they lack the grammatical knowledge), rather that they have difficulty with processing what they hear and the time that this takes them. This, coupled with demand avoidance, can lead to misunderstanding and disruption to the communication process. (Christie *et al.* 2011).

Mollie's difficulties in verbal communication mean that she appears to completely misinterpret the spoken word, which makes normal lines of communication – as you and I would know it – extremely difficult to sustain. Not to mention the demand avoidance, processing speed and the appearance of being unable to hear me at all.

Simple words of advice or a suggestion such as, 'Be careful how you hold the scissors', or 'Have you put the lids back on your pens?' are interpreted by her as being embarrassing, humiliating and implying that she is stupid. In her mind, she already knows how to hold the scissors and to put pen lids back on; she appears to interpret the instigator of these instructions as purposefully wanting to humiliate her in public. Her initial reaction to these incidents is an instant spike in anxiety, which can make her snap. If she manages to conceal the snap and press on with the role play of normality, the snap may just build up until she is free to release it as a huge 'bite' when she feels safe to do so.

Mollie may appear to have better verbal timing than other children with a more typical presentation of ASD. However, I do wonder if this, like social understanding, is at an intellectual level and simply role played by her. When she is relaxed and being herself, she constantly interrupts, talks endlessly about her own interests, has little or no interest in what the other person may want to convey and can bore the listener into an early death. Any meaningful conversation is often completely ignored and she simply turns the conversation back to role play with Blueberry Bear or goes off on a long monologue about Minecraft. Conversation with Mollie, even at the age of ten, is often based around twiddle twaddle and nothing of any real substance.

A simple and minor change in the tone or octave of voice can result in Mollie instantly feeling that she is being shouted at when she isn't. I may be frustrated, tired or simply be using a slightly firmer tone; sometimes I am completely unaware of any change in my voice but she detects it instantly. She often interprets this as being shouted at. There have been many times when I have simply put forward a suggestion, unaware that my tone of voice is any different than normal, for her to instantly react with, 'Stop yelling at me!' Again, this spikes her anxiety levels because she may feel embarrassed or under attack from the speaker. This anxiety may remain concealed beneath the veneer of normality, but it will be released in one form or another once she is with those with whom she feels safe to be herself.

A simple request or demand may be perceived by Mollie as embarrassing or as being bossed about. She may feel that by complying, she would look foolish or that she has given in and been outmanoeuvred. This is slightly different than the scissors/pen lid scenario above because we don't need to be implying that she should be careful or that she doesn't know what she is doing. Even asking an unexpected question or asking if she wants to play a well-loved game appears to put her instantly in avoidance mode because the idea/interaction has not been initiated by her. It has therefore taken her control away, which sparks an instant need for self-preservation and for her to regain that control by refusing, ignoring or distracting.

Until very recently Mollie's very advanced verbal communication was not used to share feelings or experiences or to discuss and debate. It was merely a tool that was used to direct, control and avoid situations and demands. A free-flowing reciprocal conversation was unheard of, because even asking a question that she may not have been expecting, for example 'Would you like your lunch?' would be perceived as a demand, so she would avoid answering by completely ignoring me or by talking about something completely unrelated. Verbal communication is often ignored to such an extent that we had Mollie's hearing tested. Whether this is due to processing speed or demand avoidance is not clear, but I suspect that it may be a mix of the two.

Mollie is quite good at understanding idioms and metaphors and appears to understand that these are simply a turn of phrase or a comparable way of looking at something so that it can make more sense. She does, however, appear to have difficulty understanding humour and she can take other areas of conversation literally. She can become very angry if she feels that she is being laughed at, even if we are laughing with her, rather than at her. I can remember my dad making a joke comment about Lee; it was pure banter and we were all laughing, including Lee. Mollie became very upset and told her granddad to never say those things about her dad again because they weren't true.

As with social interaction, verbal interaction is somewhat of a paradox for Mollie. Very good skills in some areas appear to mask very true difficulties in other areas.

Observations and further questions

Verbal communication is so massively misinterpreted by Mollie that it produces real confusion, anxiety and stress. She doesn't want to feel embarrassed, humiliated or shouted at. When she does experience any one or a combination of these feelings she knows that she is prone to then have either a minor or a major reaction in the form of either verbally or physically lashing out.

'Shut up', 'Stop telling me what to do', 'Stop shouting at me', or, 'Do you think I'm stupid?' are just a few of the more polite ways that she may react. These are usually very impulsive remarks blurted out with, what appears to be, great anger probably fuelled by embarrassment and anxiety. If she is deeply embarrassed, for example if a shop assistant has kindly asked her not to touch something, she may run out of the shop and try to hide somewhere. Her frustrations will then be either verbally or physically taken out on someone on whom she feels safe to do so, usually me or her dad.

Does the confusion of verbal communication, which may include misunderstanding the intention of the speaker, processing difficulties, not knowing intuitively when to speak or what about, produce the associated behaviours of controlling verbal communication by ignoring, avoiding, persistent interrupting and so on?

Is this area of communication the same as that of social interaction? Do the huge difficulties in knowing intuitively how to communicate and interpret verbal communication result in the strategies previously discussed. Is it that by controlling the communication, it becomes more predictable and more manageable for Mollie to successfully navigate without fear of failure or embarrassment?

8

Routine, Predictability, Fantasy and Obsessions

It is often said that children with PDA hate routine and thrive on novelty, which would appear to be in complete contradiction to what we would typically expect to see in a child with ASD. To a certain extent this is true: Mollie hates routine that is imposed on her by others. The novelty of a pleasant new activity can be successful in encouraging her to try something new or to engage in an activity by presenting it in a different manner. However, Mollie does need to stick to her own routine and to know what will be coming next. She appears to do this by imposing her routine on those around her and not by following a routine devised and set out by somebody else.

Because Mollie is naturally social and desperately wants to fit in, she appears to try to use routine and predictability to reduce stress levels that are spiked by the unpredictable – not knowing what will happen next and what she may get wrong. She appears to try to navigate the complex, confusing and challenging social highway by imposing her need for routine and predictability on others. Is this achieved by trying to control all areas of social interaction and communication by being in role play – in charge and in control at all times? A thought provoking suggestion was expressed by Dr Judith Gould (Director of the NAS Lorna Wing Centre), she said: 'The PDA group have been described as "hating routine and thriving on novelty". But are they imposing their routines by controlling the environment' (Judith Gould 2012 NAS/PDA Conference).

Mollie does have a rich and varied imagination, which means that she and individuals like her may fall through the 'ASD net'. However, Mollie's rich imagination and ability to role play is steeped in imitation and repetition. She will often play out the same scenario time and time again because she appears to be happy and secure knowing the outcome of the game. Mollie's Barbie and Ken, aka Corrine and Eric, can enjoy the same adventure with only slight tweaks to the story every time she plays with them. The foundation of many imaginative games can often stem from repeating what she has seen on the TV or in a movie.

As Mollie's social exposure drastically reduced her routine, her obsessions and repetition appeared to become more stereotypical of ASD. Rather than needing to control her social environment in order to provide her with routine, she became less controlling within the home and would appear happier in her own company watching back-to-back episodes of TV shows or YouTube films of people playing Minecraft, printing off picture after picture of Barbie or Power Rangers and colouring them in and so on. When she began interacting more with the outside world, we would see a drop in these typical ASD obsessions, a return to more social obsessions and a need for more control and attention from people. She currently appears to alternate between these two states.

Although Mollie became less controlling with people with whom she felt comfortable (family were fairly predictable to her), she still needed to have a strict routine of certain people for certain jobs and never the twain should meet. I am the arts and crafts person and the sensitive one who she comes to when she has something troubling her. My husband is the practical fixer required to mend things, play computer games with and be her physical protector, because he is a man and strong. Ann (who is Mollie's personal assistant funded by social services via direct payments), is the only person with whom Mollie will play Barbie and other various role play scenarios.

Mollie appears to use fantasy to reduce the stress imposed on her by the outside world. At times she can become so involved in her imaginary role play or scenarios that the edges of fantasy and reality appear blurred. Mollie has commented that when she is watching a fantasy TV series, she actually becomes a part of that show. That fantasy becomes her reality and when the series ends she feels a sense of loss at having to return to real life. When real life is too daunting, fantasy is a wonderful escape into a world that she can safely navigate. The good guy always gets the girl, the bad guy always loses and there is always a happy ending. This is a safe, calm and happy world where things never go wrong and she can safely predict what the eventual outcome will be.

She has also described how fantasy is so much more exciting than real life, because there are no vampires, warlocks, werewolves and so on in real life. She has commented that when she absorbs herself in these worlds, she feels less alone, 'I don't fit in, in this world and so I like watching these shows because the vampires and werewolves don't fit in with the normal world either. I feel like we share a connection and have something in common with each other.'

When she was younger Mollie's best friend was Blueberry Bear. Blueberry shielded her from the expectations of others and became a vehicle through whom she could communicate more freely. Blueberry became a verified family member within her own right and Mollie would refer to her as her sister. She was Mollie's constant companion – the ideal friend who never argued back or refused to do anything. Blueberry had her own bed, suitcase, wardrobe of clothes, shoes and toys. The family had to interact and handle her as if she was a real child. We could often communicate and reach Mollie by talking to Blueberry and vice versa. Blueberry would then become the fall guy for any social hiccups or mistakes. Blueberry Bear was replaced for a while with Mollie's Ipad. However following a stint at boarding school, as Mollie told us, Blueberry Bear is now back at home and very much a part of daily living again.

Mollie does have obsessions, but these can initially be harder to notice than you would typically see in a child with ASD. When Mollie was trying to navigate her way through the social highway, her obsessions would be social in nature. Her initial obsession was with me, and I was the only one who was allowed to do anything for her. She appeared to hate her father and brother and once asked me to leave them so that it would just be me and her. I essentially became a single parent because Mollie would simply not allow her dad to do anything at all, either with her or for her.

When she started school, her obsession would be directed onto another child. She would fixate on a particular child and need to be with her at all times. This could result in obsessions of hate towards other children. Perhaps this is because she feared that her beloved friend may be taken away from her. To make it through the day, she needed the company of this one special child with whom she could be herself with and whom she trusted.

I believe that the obsession with people is simply Mollie's way of keeping herself calm and protected by being with someone who can be her comfort blanket when she feels socially exposed and misunderstood. Her difficulties with socialising are made ten times worse in group situations and are more manageable on a one-to-one basis – one person is easier to predict and control than a whole group. So by reducing that group down to one primary figure, she can perhaps block the rest out and ease her anxiety. Obsessions for children with PDA can can often be social in nature as discussed by Christie *et al*.:

> Often the subjects of fixations for children with PDA tend to be social in nature and often revolve around specific individuals. This can result in blame, victimisation and harassment, which can cause real problems for peer relationships in school. (Christie *et al*. 2011, p.32)

In order for the world to make sense and feel safe Mollie became obsessed with the need to control her immediate environment and to avoid any demands made on her. The obsessive need to avoid demands exhibited by individuals with PDA is a feature that was duly noted by Professor Newson, in that 'the demand avoidant behaviour itself usually has an "obsessive feel"' (Christie *et al*. 2011, p.32).

Once social exposure was reduced, Mollie's obsessions tended to revolve around more typical topics for a child of her age and gender. However, it was the degree and the intensity with which these interests were pursued that appeared to be far from typical. Obsessions seemed to be intrinsically linked to Mollie's repetitive routines – the obsession was fulfilled by repeating it, so it became her routine.

Obsessions appear to drive repetitive routines or they can result in the need to purchase and collect stuff. She can become obsessed with an item that she has seen on TV, or in adding a particular item to her collection, and the need to acquire it becomes all-consuming. It is reminiscent of a drug addict requiring their next fix – the desire and need build in intensity until the item is purchased. Following the acquisition of the item, calm descends – for now the need driven by the obsession has been filled. The item, which she so desperately needed, will probably be played with or used for a day and then never touched again.

Observations and further questions

I think that Mollie's obsessions can also bring about routine and predictability. When she was younger she didn't really have any clear and obvious obsessions that would be typical in a child with ASD. She would like tying things up and watching reruns of Doctor Who but nothing major. The sole focus of her obsessions was around people – liking them, loathing them, controlling them or avoiding demands made by them. I suppose this obsession brought about a sense of repetition and predictability to make the social highway seem like a safer place to be.

As she withdrew, and the burden of navigating the social highway became a thing of the past, her control within the home subsided. It was as if we, her family, were now predictable enough for her no longer to feel the need to be so completely in control of us. The more control she had over her own life, the less she tried to control every aspect of ours.

Obsessions and repetitive behaviours are now less about individual people and the control of society as a whole and more based around fictional characters, scenarios, films, games and collections. However, when she spends increased periods of time interacting with family members or going out more, the more typical ASD obsessions and routines switch to obsessions with people and her control over them.

9

Summing Up the Difficulties and Empathising with Mollie

Quotes from Mollie

- 'I have a phobia of people and I don't really know who I am, what I like or who I am supposed to be.'

- 'Mum, please you can change my brain, I want a new brain I can't live the rest of my life like this.'

- 'I just want to be a normal girl that goes to school and has friends like everyone else.'

- 'When I have friends I get over excited and this pushes them away, they are frightened of me because I hit and kick and they see me scream at you. I know why I haven't got any friends but I just can't control who I am.'

- 'I am so bossy and selfish who will ever want to be with me when I get older?'

- 'I want to go out but I can't cope, even someone saying, "don't touch that," sends me into panic and then I can't control my reactions. I feel as if there are eyes watching me all the time just waiting for me to make a mistake.'

- 'It's been harder to go out since I was restrained at school. The humiliation and the shame of being held down in front of my classmates. I can see their faces now and I often imagine that it is happening all over again but this time I am on the playground and the whole school can see what is happening to me. I couldn't breathe and thought that I was going to die. Sometimes I have panic attacks even when I'm just sitting watching TV.'

- 'I am a curse on the world, a curse on my family and a curse on myself.'

Are you walking in Mollie's shoes yet? Are you empathising, understanding and recognising her difficulties? Has your image of a defiant, naughty and strong-willed child been replaced with the reality of a frightened, misunderstood and desperately unhappy child whose self-esteem has been crushed and who is taunted on a daily basis by an outside world that she desperately wants to be a part of?

Mollie does not exhibit the behaviour typified in the diagnostic criteria for PDA, because she is strong-willed, naughty and in need of a firm hand. She exhibits this behaviour due to the same level of difficulties with 'autistic-like traits' as other individuals with ASD, that is, difficulties associated with social interaction, social communication, social imagination (which can appear strong but may be lacking in depth) and difficulties with peers.

As an extra layer of complexity, she also experiences difficulties with anti-social behaviour, a lack of pro-social behaviour and higher levels of emotional problems than individuals with a more typical presentation of ASD.

Put all of these difficulties in a mixing pot and stir them up, carefully combining all of the ingredients. Leave the mixture fully exposed to the outside world for approximately 18 months and then you may see the ingredients gradually begin to transform into the PDA profile. The longer the ingredients are left exposed to the outside world, the more extreme, obvious and severe that PDA profile may become. This appears to be a unique mixture of ingredients; when combined they seem to transform into a unique profile: the PDA profile.

In Mollie's particular case, the continued exposure to the outside world caused such a dramatic and extreme reaction to her internal ingredients/makeup that she simply couldn't control the rapid metamorphosis that began to occur. Frightened, confused, anxious and unable to understand or stop what was happening to her, she ran away and hid from the outside world. She must have felt that she had no other choice but to hide and return to the safety of an impenetrable cocoon, home!

I hope that your eyes and imagination have been opened and that you can think outside of the box of traditional behaviour modification, because those strategies have no place in my world. Mollie is not naughty and did not need to be made to 'fit in'. What she needed was for us to adapt our behaviours towards her. We needed to provide Mollie with an environment where she could heal, learn, understand and feel free to be herself. Then we could gradually teach her how to cope with exposure to the outside world and how to adapt and moderate her less desirable or more unacceptable behaviours.

You may now be ready to understand the very radical and unorthodox strategies and parenting style that have been required to save my little girl and our family from complete destruction.

The strategies that we have employed have had to be extreme but, in light of what you have read, I do hope that they will make sense.

But before we start on strategies, let's first have a quick look at what Mollie may perceive as being a 'demand that she has an anxiety-driven need to avoid' and how this can quickly escalate into a meltdown. It may be wider reaching and more encompassing than you imagine!

Part 4

Breaking the
PDA Cycle

10

The Cycle of Demand, Control, Avoidance and Meltdown

Normal, everyday living is loaded with demands for Mollie – many of them are obvious, some are so subtle that we may not even realise that she would perceive them as a demand and some are invisible to us because they are the silent demands made by Mollie herself or by the unspoken rules and expectations of society.

Let's have a look at how these demands fall into these different categories so that we understand the variety of demands that Mollie is exposed to and therefore tries to avoid on a daily basis.

The obvious and direct demand

- Get up, get dressed, brush your teeth, brush your hair and so on.
- Tidy your toys up.
- Time for bed.
- Wash your hands.

- Say please, say thank you.
- Look at this.
- Don't do that.
- Be quiet.
- Stop interrupting me.
- Stand in a line.
- Sit down for carpet time.

The subtle and general demand

- Simply expecting a response to a question.
- Suggesting an activity that I know that Mollie enjoys.
- Leaving the house, even if it is for a fun activity.
- Advising Mollie on how to do something safely.
- Trying to explain the instructions of a game, i.e. to teach Mollie.
- Attending school.
- Someone else's suggestion to go on a fun day out.
- Following someone else's timetable for the day.
- Walking the same way or at the same pace as her parents.

The invisible demand

- Sleeping to a timescale that is perceived to be acceptable by society, i.e. awake in the day and asleep at night.
- Fitting into specific gender roles created by either nature or nurture.

- The need for perfection and for everything to go to plan for a special event such as a birthday or Christmas.

- Wanting a drink or to change the TV channel becomes a demand on herself, which can leave Mollie unable to complete the simplest of tasks on her own (this may explain why Mollie is always shouting at me to do every little thing for her).

This is only a short list, but I hope it allows you to see how anything and everything can be interpreted as a demand and how this is pervasive through all areas of Mollie's life.

Mollie has said to me that avoiding demands is instinctive – it is simply part of her internal makeup and something that she often does without even thinking about it. For her, avoiding demands and avoiding fitting into society's rules are what comes naturally. Therefore, making her behave in a way that she isn't naturally hardwired or programmed to do means that she naturally and instinctively puts up a wall of resistance.

The unpredictability of life means that she is already in a heightened sense of alert and perpetual panic because she doesn't know what demands will be made of her. Complying with demands requires her not to be herself so she avoids doing this at all costs. When she can't be her natural self or when this is threatened, she panics, her anxieties rise and she can rapidly go into free fall, otherwise known as a meltdown.

First-line strategies that Mollie uses

Ignoring or playing deaf is a familiar first line of defence to avoid immediate compliance. It is as if ignoring gives Mollie breathing space to think of her next move. Or she may simply need time to process the request and comply once she feels that the initial demand has been diluted by time.

Switching to a different topic in order to distract me from my initial request is also a common strategy, for example asking Mollie to brush her teeth may be answered with, 'I'm on episode 56 of *Pokémon* now and I only have 300 more to watch.'

She may promise to do whatever is being asked of her 'in a minute' or 'when I've finished this' or offer a list of imaginary reasons why something can't be done, such as 'I can't because my arms are aching, my legs are sore, my body doesn't work.'

Mollie may negotiate with me and offer to comply only after I have done something first, for example 'I'll do it if you buy me this toy', or 'If you do arts and crafts with me I will do it after.' She may put her hands over her ears and drown out requests and demands by simultaneously singing songs. Or she may bombard me with repeated questions to avoid the demand being repeated.

Any deals that are made are likely to be reneged on and the goalposts will be repeatedly moved. If I carry on asking and become more forceful, Mollie's anxiety and resistance can increase and the strategies may move to level two.

Level two strategies that Mollie uses

Shock tactics may be employed in an effort to get rid of me and bring a halt to the demand, such as shouting at me to, 'shut up', or 'f**k off', or giving me a controlled hit or kick or a combination of both.

She may start to throw things at me, empty the contents of drawers onto the floor while shouting at me to, 'F**k off you fat bitch.' At this stage she is still in control of her behaviour, if not her rising anxiety, and these are controlled actions aimed at making me to stop pushing the demand.

When she was younger, she would remove her clothes, urinate on the floor or do both. This tactic was particularly useful if she wanted to shock a visitor into leaving, particularly Jake's friends. This type of behaviour was more prevalent at around the age of seven and fortunately we do not see it now.

If I continue to push the demand and don't act upon these warning signs, her anxiety levels will continue to escalate and she may go into a full meltdown, best seen as a panic attack. This is the stage where all her actions and behaviour are no longer within her control – she is now effectively in free fall!

How Mollie behaves during a meltdown

A meltdown is like an explosion of anxiety and frustration being released in one surge of energy. By this stage, Mollie is no longer in control of her actions. She may repeatedly lash out at me, both physically and verbally, often requiring me to try to restrain her to stop the repeated blows or to adopt a position that protects me from them.

The trashing of the house is no longer controlled – anything and everything in sight is thrown, and she may need restraining to prevent her from breaking windows or throwing objects that could really hurt someone. This level of meltdown can last for hours and is exhausting for all concerned.

Following the meltdown, Mollie may remain very angry, anxious, stressed or confused and she may need space or be very upset and require a cuddle. The after-effects of the meltdown can simmer away under the surface for hours or even a few days, and during this time she is extremely susceptible to a quick and rapid increase to meltdown level again.

If Mollie is very anxious or has already coped with a lot of demands, the reaction time from demand to meltdown can be instantaneous with no obvious triggers. She can go from 0 to 60 in seconds, cutting out the steady build-up of level one and level two.

Triggers for a meltdown

A demand being pushed on Mollie, especially if she is being threatened with a punishment or bribed with a reward, can trigger a meltdown. We don't do this now but our lack of understanding meant that in the past we did.

If Mollie feels a loss of control when her needs, orders or requests are not complied with, or if she feels ignored and that others are receiving more attention than her, this can produce challenging behaviours that can quickly escalate into a meltdown.

She may be experiencing already high anxiety levels caused by a completely unrelated person or situation, that day or on a previous day, which can cause her tolerance for any new demands to be extremely low.

Being exposed to too much sensory stimuli or social exposure, for example noise, supermarkets, smells and so on, can increase anxiety levels to the point of meltdown especially if demands are then loaded on top.

Transitions are also another massive trigger for meltdowns if they aren't handled sensitively. The demand to leave somewhere, coupled with knowing that the fun will be continuing without her, can cause Mollie a huge amount of anxiety.

In short, not feeling in full control of herself, her immediate environment and the people in it can lead to challenging behaviour that can quickly escalate into a meltdown.

How I deal with a meltdown

If I see the signs of a meltdown approaching, I may have time to distract Mollie or to immediately empathise about whatever has caused her the upset. This may soothe her and bring anxiety down.

I do not try to stop the natural progress of a meltdown by using the threat of rewards or punishments; I simply allow it to run its natural course while also being there for her. Trying to stop it by exerting control, and therefore insinuating that Mollie has control of her own rising anxiety levels, is likely to intensify and prolong the meltdown.

The trick for us has been to assist Mollie through her meltdowns by allowing her to have a certain amount of self-expression in order to release her internal pressure cooker. We have found that by allowing her to trash things, within reason, this release, without any parental intervention, can prevent the next level from occurring. I do not intervene or try to rationalise or negotiate with her unless she is putting either herself or someone else at risk.

I always endeavour to give her as much space and freedom of expression as she requires during a meltdown, while at the same time keeping a safe distance so that she doesn't feel that I am watching her every move.

I don't consider that the damage of property requires my intervention if it is damage that can be tided away or cleaned up, such as drawers being emptied or toy boxes turned over. I do, however, stop the throwing of breakables or windows being smashed. I try to remain quiet, calm and vigilant. If the meltdown progresses to physical violence or activities that could be a health and safety risk then I do, only at this point, physically intervene.

We have found that this approach to meltdowns has helped to lower their intensity and shorten their duration. This does not always work, and if Mollie wants something in particular that we have denied, for example to control her brother's interactions with friends, then we often have to go through hours of meltdowns; her brother's emotional well-being is one of the few areas not open to negotiation. I never, ever punish a meltdown either during or following the incident.

As she calms down I may ask her if she wants a hug, express empathy, explain that I understand why she is so upset and reassure her that she is not in trouble and that she is deeply loved. I will wait for her to signal to me that she is now calm enough for me to physically approach her and that she is ready to engage with me.

We found that dealing with meltdowns in this way meant that they gradually became far more manageable and less explosive. Eventually we reached the idyllic situation of Mollie no longer having these intense meltdowns. However, this was due to a variety of factors, which shall be revealed throughout the book, and we remain prepared for their return.

11

Strategies that Help Mollie Feel in Control

So, if we combine the difficulties that Mollie experiences around social interaction, social communication, emotional issues, impulsiveness and demands, accompanied by the need for her own repetitive routines, sensory issues and obsessions, it starts to become clear why these difficulties cause such complex and extreme behaviours. The profile of PDA begins to make sense and the use of PDA strategies tailored to meet Mollie's specific needs begins to become tangible, rather than just something we apply because it appears to bring about successful results, without actually understanding why.

As with any other autism spectrum disorder, children with PDA are on a spectrum. Some may be severely affected by their difficulties and require extreme intervention, and some may be mildly affected thus requiring minimal intervention.

With the correct support and implementation of basic strategies, some children may cope quite well in life and at school. They may be more tolerant of demands and rules than another child with PDA, so it may be unnecessary to make radical changes.

Bearing in mind that these children are on a spectrum, here are the PDA strategies combined with our own strategies and interventions that we have used for Mollie. I do consider Mollie to have a very extreme presentation of PDA due to very high levels of anxiety. I think that this is typified by her persistent school refusal from the age of six eventually leading to a complete inability to continue with school. Even though she had excellent support and her needs were being met by the LEA, she still suffered with extreme anxiety, which ultimately led to extreme and challenging behaviour. Mollie's anxieties became so high and her fears of the outside world were so intense that for long periods of time she became unable to leave her own home.

How we applied PDA strategies to Mollie

The defining diagnostic criterion for PDA is an anxiety-driven need to avoid the demands of everyday life and to be in control at all times. The strategies recommended by the Elizabeth Newson Centre, the PDA Society and the book *Understanding Pathological Demand Avoidance Syndrome in Children* (Christie *et al.* 2011) suggest trying to reduce the anxiety of everyday demands to help the child feel in control, but also to be flexible and to slightly increase demands on days when the child appears more able to tolerate them. This is how we personally applied those strategies to Mollie, combined with our own interventions, which we tailored to meet Mollie's needs and her complexity.

Our non-negotiable boundaries

By the time Mollie was seven, we were having such a difficult time; her anxiety and behaviour had accelerated to such a high level that we decided to have as few non-negotiable boundaries as possible. Our non-negotiable boundaries were enforced and we remained firm and stood our ground.

Even maintaining these few boundaries was exhausting, involved hours of meltdowns and never served to change her behaviour in the short term. Maintaining these boundaries was extremely important and took all of our strength, patience and resolve. It was a little bit like doing a risk assessment on what was really important to us and where our energies needed to be used. Everything else was up for negotiation, discussion or compromise.

If Mollie was a danger to herself or anybody else then we would intervene to stop the dangerous behaviour or actions. Believe me, when Mollie was younger, just implementing health and safety boundaries became a huge task.

Jake's emotional well-being and him having a safe private place to interact with his friends was and still is of paramount importance to us. Mollie continually disrupting his interactions with friends, becoming physically or verbally abusive to him or trying to control him excessively to the point of him becoming extremely stressed were all situations that we would act on. Mollie would either be tempted into another activity with an adult or, if this didn't produce the desired result, she would be physically removed from his room.

If Mollie was hurting or upsetting other children, either in the home, during play dates or in the street, then this was also acted on. Mollie would be brought inside or, if the incident was occurring inside the house, the other child would be taken home.

Strategies

- *We always try to phrase demands in a ways that offer Mollie choices and we are always prepared to negotiate or back down completely:* Phrasing a request in a way that invites Mollie to help solve a problem can also be a useful tool to encourage her involvement. We tried to give Mollie the balance of control within parameters that we could comfortably meet.

  - Would you like to get dressed now or later on?

  - I've made a big list of games that we can play – would you like to choose one?

  - Your dinner is ready. Where would you like to eat it – at the table, at your computer or in front of the TV?

  - We have had a new carpet and I really would like to try and keep it clean. I really don't mind if you keep your shoes on but I would be so grateful if you could take them off before you go into the lounge. It really is up to you though.

  - I'm really stuck on this jigsaw, is there any chance that you can help me?

  - If bedtime was at 9.00pm, we would tell Mollie that bedtime was at 8.00pm and then allow her to negotiate with us so that, when we settled at somewhere between 8.00pm and 9.00pm, she felt that she had the final say.

  - Would you like to go to the cinema? You can choose the film, the day and the time?

  - Do you want to brush your teeth before or after breakfast?

- What night this week would you like to take a bath or a shower?

This basic strategy of choice could be very hit and miss with Mollie. She would often pre-empt what we were trying to achieve and outwit us at our own game. Some days it would bring about the desired result and on others it would fail miserably. However, this strategy is basic, generic and only a very small cog in a large wheel. As her overall level of anxiety came down due to the combination of strategies used, this way of offering choices to Mollie did become more successful.

- *We adopt a tone or style of voice that Mollie finds non-threatening:* Mollie appears to completely misunderstand verbal communication and may interpret everything as being a demand, being shouted out or inferring that she must be stupid. We try to adopt either a 'children's TV presenter' persona when we are interacting with her – all light, bubbly and excitable – or a very soft, slow and calm tone. She appears to find this less threatening than a more normal delivery of speech. The style and tone that you may need to adopt will depend on what your child finds the least threatening or patronising.

- *We give our child as much control as we can over her own environment, including control over me, and I only intervene if I feel that it is a safeguarding issue:* Allowing myself to become totally subservient to Mollie's whims wasn't easy and there were consequences for my own mental health. However, it was better than enduring the meltdowns, which only served to perpetuate the problem. This is what she needed, at that time, to keep her anxiety levels on an even keel. In time, when she was in a better place mentally, we would help her to release some of that control.

We now experience periods when Mollie completely relaxes her control over me and occupies herself for a long time. There can be times when she requires complete control over me, especially during events that spike anxiety or excitement, like Christmas or birthdays. I tolerate as much control as I can take, but there are times when I have to say enough is enough and walk through the eye of the 'Mollie storm'.

- *We try to be flexible and go with the flow – successful achievements on one day (when tolerance for demands is high) may not be achievable on another day (when tolerance for demands is low) and expectations have to be adjusted accordingly:* The one thing that is certain about PDA is the unpredictability and uncertainty of how Mollie will cope with and respond to demands on any given day. We may have days of relatively calm behaviour when demands are readily accepted and complied with followed by days of complete refusal and meltdowns. Strategies that are successful on one day could fail miserably on the next day.

  On days of calm, when anxieties are low, we enjoy the freedom that this extra tolerance for demands affords us. On days of high anxiety and stress, we reduce and strip back the demands and the expectations placed on Mollie to a level that she can cope with. There are many factors that can alter Mollie's tolerance for demands at any given moment, which I shall discuss later.

- *We try to recognise the subtle clues that may indicate that tolerance is low, and allow Mollie the space that she needs and reduce our expectations for compliance:* This can change by the minute, never mind by the day. We have become highly attuned to identifying the subtle clues and triggers that indicate that Mollie is not coping. The key is knowing when we can gently push and when we needed to pull back. A delayed response to a question, Mollie appearing agitated and snapping quickly at remarks or Mollie going into manic excitement were and still are possible indicators that it is best to proceed with caution and reduce demands to an absolute minimum.

- *Rewards, consequences, sticker charts and so on may produce some short-term success, possibly due to the novelty factor:* However if they are used long term they are generally unsuccessful for Mollie and often only serve to make a bad situation even worse. A reward or consequence can make Mollie feel less in control because it gives me the balance of power with the carrot or stick. The reward or consequence can feel very unjust if Mollie simply *can't* rather than *won't*. Mollie may, quiet rightly, interpret the use of rewards and consequences as being manipulated, bribed and blackmailed by the person instigating them. This reduces her control over the situation and can anger her, because, in her eyes, I am trying underhand tactics. I never underestimate Mollie's ability to completely and totally see through many of the tactics I may use to try to promote compliance.

- *We try to use surprise rewards that haven't been used to promote compliance:* Surprise rewards as a natural consequence of behaviour won't necessarily promote future compliance but will give Mollie a sense of well-being and a feel-good factor. For example, saying, 'Thank you so much for helping me tidy up – now I have got more time to play on the computer with you.' Tidying up has given Mollie a reward but without the sense of bribery, manipulation or praise for complying, which may make Mollie feel that she has given in and therefore been outmanoeuvred.

- *The same can be said for consequences, so we tend to use natural consequences:* Threatening Mollie with a consequence or giving her a consequence for bad behaviour does nothing to solve the root cause of the issue. It only increases her anger and anxiety, lowers her self-esteem and causes her even more underlying resentment.

  A lot of behaviour is driven by complex difficulties causing huge anxiety and is not within her control. Dishing out a consequence does not suddenly mean that she will gain control of her anxiety-driven behaviour anymore than punishing a child in a wheelchair will promote walking.

  However, a natural consequence that does not involve yielding the axe over her may help in certain areas, for example, 'I understand that you hate wearing a seatbelt but we can't leave until you are nice and safe because it is the law.' The natural consequence is that we can't leave until the demand has been complied with.

- *There need to be as few boundaries as possible and ideally either disguised or blamed on a higher power:* Many boundaries tend to be more readily accepted by Mollie if they are either disguised or enforced because they are the law, health and safety requirements and so on. For example, the health and safety rules at the local pool may specify that no running is allowed at poolside so that children don't fall and hurt themselves. Simply highlighting a no running poster to Mollie may be more productive than directly telling her not to run at the poolside. After all, it isn't my rule, but one that is coming from a higher power.

When Mollie used to play outside and we wanted her to be in for a certain time, we attempted to disguise this demand. We would say that we needed her to be in by 8.00pm because the younger children in the street need it to be quiet so that they could go to sleep. She always appeared to accept this as a justified reason.

- *If Mollie is having a bad day and is very 'spiky' then Blueberry Bear can be a useful ally:* We embraced Blueberry and used her to our advantage, making the most of the fantasy world that Mollie often drifts into. Communicating through Blueberry could deflect and make Mollie more amenable to the demand. The demand was from Blueberry, so Mollie was not losing any control by complying. Or if the demand has been made by Blueberry, she may deem that complying with a bear isn't too big a deal. Mollie would often feel more comfortable expressing feelings and concerns through Blueberry.

- *We empathise with Mollie if someone or something has upset her:* We have learned that we get nowhere by trying to point out the other side of the coin, other than potentially to push her towards a meltdown. The peak of upset and anxiety is not the time to try and make Mollie see the bigger picture or the other person's point of view. For the sake of avoiding the situation escalating, we simply agree, empathise and maybe inject a spark of humour aimed at undermining the culprit. The aim is to de-escalate and salvage a potentially combustible situation.

Mollie needs to feel that we are on her side and have her back. The time to teach empathy will come at a later date. My husband and I work as a team of good cop/bad cop and the roles are interchangeable depending on which one of us has upset Mollie. If Lee has upset her, I may say, 'Oh Mollie, I totally agree with you but you know what a dumpty your dad can be, I really don't know how we both put up with him.' This is a cue for him to respond with humour, 'I don't know how you dare say such things about me,' with a wry grin. Straight away the huge spike in the anxiety monitor drops and the meltdown is stopped in its tracks. We then work on helping Mollie to cope with whatever has caused the spike in behaviour and come up with strategies at a calmer time.

- *Routine and structure tend not to work with Mollie unless they are her own:* We cannot impose our routine and structure on Mollie. If we need to engage her or encourage compliance, we find that an armoury of different and novel strategies is a far more successful way of achieving our objective.

  However, Mollie does need to have her own routine and structure, which she will try to impose on others when she is interacting socially. She may have her own fixed idea of what the events of each day will hold and she can become extremely stressed and anxious if this is not facilitated. We do try to facilitate her needs and the expectations because we realise how important her routine is to her.

  It is difficult to constantly meet Mollie's immediate needs at only a moment's notice. However, I do try to remember that it may not be a moment's notice to her; she may have been planning the day's events well in advance but simply not thought to communicate this to me. The thought of what she had planned not actually being fulfilled probably feels catastrophic to her. However inconvenient or annoying it is to have to drop everything at a moment's notice in order to meet Mollie's demand, I have found that complying can, in the long run, be the quickest and easiest option.

A meltdown may last far longer and prove to be far more stressful than just going along with what Mollie may need at any given moment. We are currently trying to help Mollie to understand why it is difficult for us always to be on standby and how this can affect us. As she matures, I hope we may be able to work on strategies to help her cope with not being able to have everything immediately.

- *When situations occur that we are not happy with, we do not try and deal with them immediately:* Every so often we may unexpectedly find ourselves in uncharted territory where the options are to go with flow, sometimes against our better judgement, or a meltdown. As long as no one's health and safety is at risk, we tend to go with the flow in order to avoid the meltdown and reflect after the event on how we can avoid this happening again.

An example of this is the time that my parents first took Mollie swimming. My poor dad and Mollie jumped in the pool at 2.00pm and when it was time to get out she point-blank refused and wanted to stay until the pool closed at 6.00pm. He was cold and bored but he could not get her to come out and pushing her to comply was obviously resulting in high anxiety and the possibility of a meltdown.

As your child gets older, scooping them up and physically removing them ceases to be an option. So my dad made the wise decision to just grin and bear it and then to think how he could avoid the same situation happening next time they went.

We discussed the situation at home and we negotiated with Mollie a suitable amount of time to stay in the pool. We started off by offering an hour and let her barter with her granddad until an agreed time of two hours had been reached. With this in mind, the next time he took her swimming he arrived at 4.00pm so that once the two hours was completed the pool would be closing, which would make it easier for her to leave. The problem of leaving the pool never happened again.

- *Humour can be a really useful tool to defuse a situation, but it needs to be used with caution:* If Mollie feels that we are laughing at her then this can make matters worse. However, encouraging her to laugh at someone else's predicament can help to distract her from the original source of her upset. This is an area where Blueberry Bear can come into her own. If we can manipulate Blueberry to do something funny – pull a funny face or do something cheeky like break wind – this can distract her enough to embark on a game with Blueberry.

- *We allow and allocate extra time so that Mollie does not feel pressured by time constraints, which ultimately become another demand:* Mollie may become even more agitated and stressed if we push her to 'hurry up' because we are running late. Not only does this reinforce the demand, but she also picks up on our stress, which in turn increases hers. In order to help with this problem, we drastically reduced our daily expectations to a bare minimum allowing huge amounts of time for the smallest of tasks.

This removes the pressure of everything being done within a time constraint. For example, if Mollie is having a bath she can take as much or as little time as she wishes because there is nothing else predetermining the timescale of the bath.

It can take between one and one-and-a-half hours for her to transition from waking up to coming downstairs. Therefore, except for in exceptional circumstances, we only arrange to do things in an afternoon. This removes the pressure of a time limit within which to get up and get ready. Mollie tends to take ten times as long as a neurotypical child to do anything, so our daily lives have to allow for this fact.

- *We are careful with what we do and don't praise Mollie for:* I always praise Mollie for anything that she has done under her own steam that she is obviously pleased and relaxed about. I tend to intuitively know when she would like to be praised for something by reading her body language and demeanour. If she has drawn a lovely picture or made a wonderful model on her own and through her own instigation I will say what a lovely job she has done.

  If she has complied with something that was initially suggested by me, like having a bath or brushing her teeth, I never praise her, because this can be interpreted as me blowing my own trumpet because she has complied. Some children rip up their own work in school; this may be because any work completed in school is usually done under duress and at the instigation of someone else.

  At home, fun activities are usually self-motivated, so we can praise her. However, if Mollie complies with a demand that usually prompts avoidance we just remain silent and act as if it hasn't happened. I would never make a fuss and praise Mollie for washing her hair, because that would simply reduce the possibility of her ever doing it again!

- *We try to pick the right time to talk to Mollie and make it as relaxed as possible:* With the correct strategies and in the right environment, Mollie, especially as she's grown older, has begun to open up to me and has occasionally been prepared to discuss her feelings.

  We don't try to discuss situations in the middle of a meltdown when Mollie is stressed, anxious or engrossed in a special interest. I have found that a good time to talk is when we are both relaxed and chilled, usually just before we go to sleep or when she wakes up. Mollie currently still sleeps with me and so these are times of little distraction, warmth, comfort and safety. To help Mollie feel relaxed and not under pressure from the demands of a conversation, I will always start by saying, 'Mollie can I ask you a question or discuss something with you? It is okay if not, I just thought that I would ask.' Mollie's response will then let me know if this is going to be a good time or not.

  We may discuss how she is feeling or strategies to help her leave the house or negotiate and come to a mutually satisfactory conclusion regarding a problem that may have popped up during the week and so on. This is when I can learn the most and make the most headway with my child.

I could go on and on, but I hope you get the picture. This method of communication and management needed to become second nature and be used consistently in order to gradually reduce stress and anxiety levels with regard to demands whether real or perceived. Changes did not happen overnight, because undoing the damage, implementing a completely different style of parenting and then waiting for those changes to make a tangible difference to Mollie's anxiety levels all took time.

12

Strategies for Other Areas of Difficulty

Sensory Issues, Sleep, Transitions, Obsessions and More

The other areas of difficulty that I have outlined below and the strategies that we use for Mollie are the ones that have proved to be the most successful for Mollie and our family. I am not a professional and my experience of PDA is in relation to one child only but this is how we navigated other areas of difficulty.

Sensory processing disorder

This is a term used to describe a condition that occurs when an individual's ability to accurately process sensory stimuli appears to not function correctly. Sensory input may be processed to strongly or not strongly enough. In order to regulate these dysfunctional inputs individuals may actively seek or avoid certain sensory stimuli in order to address the balance. I think that it is commonly agreed that most, if not all, individuals on the spectrum will have sensory issues to one degree or another.

This is such a large topic that it is too complex to give it justice in this book. I would advise that you study this area in its entirety; there is plenty of information about sensory issues on the internet and in published books dedicated entirely to this subject.

In short there are seven senses and an individual may be under sensitive (hyposensitive) or over sensitive (hypersensitive) in any of these areas. In some cases an individual may be both over and under sensitive at the same time meaning that a light touch can be uncomfortable but at the same time a firm hug may be comforting. Quiet and loud noises may be processed by the brain at the same volume, meaning that there may be no gentle background noise but only constant and overpowering loud foreground noise which can be overwhelming to the individual.

So in conjunction with the difficulties that Mollie already faces in relation to everyday socialising she also has difficulties with processing her senses. Clothes may itch and irritate, and noises may bombard the brain at the same volume. Visual stimuli may cause very hyperactive behaviour and headaches when the system becomes overloaded while at the same time cause problems with reading and writing when the opposite occurs. Below are examples of behaviours that may indicate difficulties with the senses.

Auditory

- *Signs of hypersensitivity*: may cover ears in noisy places, easily startled by noises, may appear uncomfortable or distracted by sounds not noticed by others, for example, hairdryer, flushing toilet, fan, hand dryer in public toilets.

- *Signs of hyposensitivity*: may not respond to verbal cues, requires constant noise or loud music, may often require things repeating.

Visual

- *Signs of hypersensitivity*: may find brightly lit rooms or sunny days uncomfortable, can become over-stimulated with lots of visual stimuli, for example, supermarkets or brightly coloured rooms.

- *Signs of hyposensitivity*: may have difficulty controlling the eye movements and tracking objects. This may produce difficulty of a dyslexia nature, for example, letters moving around the page, difficulty copying from a whiteboard and difficulty reading.

Oral

- *Signs of hypersensitivity*: may dislike toothpaste and brushing their teeth, may be a very picky eater and gag on certain textures and tastes.

- *Signs of hyposensitivity*: may lick and chew inedible objects, may have a preference for strong flavoured or spicy food.

Smell

- *Signs of hypersensitivity*: may appear very distressed at certain smells, smells that are not normally noticed by others may be overpowering, may only eat food that they like the smell of.

- *Signs of hyposensitivity:* may smell anything and everything or appear oblivious to strong odours.

Vestibular (the sense of movement)

- *Signs of hypersensitivity:* may avoid swings, slides and any equipment that generates movement, may not like sudden movements or being held upside down or playfully tossed in the air.

- *Signs of hyposensitivity:* may seek out constant movement in the form of twirling, bouncing or swinging, may be very active and always on the go, may appear to be a thrill seeker.

Proprioceptive (the sense of 'position' of your body in space and the input from muscles and joints to the brain)

- *Signs of under-responsiveness:* may love bear hugs, appear very heavy-footed and love play fighting, may love tight clothing and the feeling of something heavy, for example, a weighted blanket or a heavy backpack. The individual may have difficulty in applying the correct amount of pressure, which may result in pushing too hard and breaking things, for example too much pressure when writing may result in the paper being torn or the pencil frequently snapping.

- *Signs of over responsiveness:* may have difficulty knowing where their body is in relation to the space around them, may bump into objects or people and appear to be clumsy or appear to be under your feet or in your way.

Tactile

- *Signs of hypersensitivity*: may be highly sensitive to clothing, certain textures, labels and seams in socks to name but a few, may be highly uncomfortable and irritated, may flinch away from hugs, cuddles or kisses and avoid baths or showers, may have a very low threshold for pain, may dislike the feeling of wearing shoes and prefer lightweight and open-toed footwear.

- *Signs of hyposensitivity*: may seek out messy play and not realise or care if hands are messy or dirty, can have a very high threshold for pain and may even have serious accidents but not even flinch, may sensory seek by touching everything and anything.[1]

As I said, this topic is extremely complex and really can't be covered in its entirety in this book, but here are a few of the common strategies that many individuals may adopt to help with some areas of sensory processing disorder.

- Wearing sunglasses in shops or outdoors to subdue visual stimuli.

- For dyslexia or Irlen syndrome, there are now several opticians that offer unique, individually tailored tinted lenses, which greatly reduce the effects of visual stimuli.

- Removing labels from clothes, buying seamless socks and wearing shoes that are open and comfortable.

- Trampolines and peanut balls are great for releasing excess energy or for those who are sensory seeking movement.

- Chewy toys are great for the oral sensory seekers.

---

1   This information has been adapted from www.sensory-processing-disorder.com.

- Always taking a packed lunch of items that your child can eat if you are going out.

- Ear protectors or headphones with music can protect from too many auditory stimuli.

- Weighted blankets can provide deep pressure for those who seek a firm touch or may help to reduce fidgeting in those who have difficulty in keeping still.

- A scented candle or something similar could help distract those unpleasant smells.

- Going to shops in the evening when the hustle and bustle of the peak flow has calmed down could be a practical alternative to the busy, over-stimulating times.[2]

Sleep

A huge issue for Mollie, which has been going on for several years, is getting her to go to bed and go to sleep. This appears to be an extremely common area of difficulty in children with learning difficulties, especially in those with autism.

Possible reasons for sleep avoidance

There may be multiple reasons for why Mollie finds going to bed and going to sleep so difficult. For one, going to bed is a complex transition loaded with demands and expectations.

Bedtime and going to sleep is a transition where one day ends and another one begins, and Mollie really struggles with transitions. The present day is comfortable

---

2   A further source of information on sensory issues in autism is: www.autism.org.uk/living-with-autism/understanding-behaviour/the-sensory-world-of-autism.

and under control but the next day is uncertain and unknown territory. Perhaps staying awake is a way of delaying the next day. This may be even more relevant if the next day involves doing something extremely stressful, such as attending school. As we all know, the quicker we fall asleep, the quicker the next day arrives.

Going to sleep while the house stays awake means that Mollie may experience a sense of loss of control over what interactions continue while she sleeps. Added to this may be the additional fear of not being able to control her dreams. Sleep is the one area where all control is lost!

The need to continue with an obsession, for example playing a game or watching TV, may override the ability to stop and transition to bed. Boredom can be another issue, because a quick, active and hyperactive mind may just not be able to settle down enough for sleep and lying awake is boring and difficult to deal with. Perhaps the quietness and solitude of a sleeping house is when Mollie is at her most relaxed and this is why staying awake and pursuing her interests during this period is so appealing to her.

Finally, there is always the possibility that Mollie may simply be frightened and have phobias, making bed a very scary place to be.

Basic generic strategies that we have tried over the years have delivered us varying amounts of success or, in some cases, complete failure. Previous successes, or even failures, could always be revisited or rotated. What worked for a few months last year while it was a novel idea, may well work again a few months down the line.

Actually getting Mollie up the stairs can be the hardest part, so we found it helpful to allow Mollie to devise a sleep routine of her own, within parameters of what we found acceptable. Letting her feel in control of her bedtime would, at times, be a successful strategy.

The fewer demands there are around bedtime, the better, so if it meant no teeth brushing or refusing to wear pyjamas, we let these small things go if we were going to win the bigger battle of bed and sleep.

We tried to make her bedroom as friendly, inviting, calm and as restful as possible. We had calming lava lamps in her room and she would have the option of an audio book or soft music to give her something to focus on to aid the boredom of trying to fall asleep.

At times Mollie appeared to very scared about staying upstairs on her own, so we would stay with her and cuddle her while she fell asleep and then return downstairs.

I used to play the name game with Mollie and occasionally we still play it. It consists of naming six girls' names beginning with A and then six beginning with B, and we would work our way through the alphabet. Often she wouldn't play at all but seemed to find the sound of my voice soothing.

We also managed to get Mollie prescribed melatonin, which is a natural remedy that prepares the mind and body for sleep. However, it only tends to work if the individual taking the melatonin is actively trying to induce sleep rather than avoid it. Mollie would sometimes take it and go to sleep, sometimes takes it and stay awake or sometimes refuse to take it at all.

During the past four years we have tried all of these strategies and they have all worked at different times, but success has never been long term and we have had to constantly chop and change the routine. Ultimately, the only person who actually had full control of when or where Mollie would sleep was Mollie herself. Resistance was futile – hour after hour of meltdowns into the early hours of the morning were not acceptable to us, especially as the meltdowns or firm stance never produced the desired change. Instead, we looked at how to manage the situation in a way that produced the least stress for all of us.

Mollie's sleep story

When Mollie was about six years old and we first started experiencing issues with getting her to go to bed, it was because she couldn't tear herself away from the TV. She would only go upstairs if she could go into her brother's room and watch TV there. This did work for a period of time, and she would watch TV or a film and be happy to turn the TV off and go to sleep when we asked her. We treated her to a TV for her room and she would happily watch a film, switch off and go to sleep.

As the novelty wore off or the realisation that she was complying sunk in – or perhaps a mixture of the two occurred – the difficulties started again. Actually getting her upstairs in the first place took longer and longer with one delay tactic after another. Once upstairs, I would be held captive with one request after another in order to prevent me from going back downstairs. We would repeatedly be called to fetch this and fetch that and would eventually still be trying to settle her down into the early hours of the morning. Even the TV could no longer hold her attention and keep her in bed. Instead, she delighted in annoying everyone else and keeping them awake by using a variety of strategies within her armoury.

Then we tried lavender oil, talking books (thinking that they would be less stimulating than the TV), weighted blankets and a pillow with an inbuilt MP3 player on to which we downloaded soothing music. All these methods failed. She would run around the house into the wee hours and it was not uncommon for me to be woken up by a punch to the face.

When we moved house, she wouldn't even go up to bed, let alone stay there for any length of time, so we tried a different approach. During this stage she was extremely hyperactive and would be bouncing of the ceiling day and night. With gentle persuasion, she began a routine of watching a film with her dad every night on the sofa until she fell asleep and then we would carry her upstairs. Sometimes it would take two or three films, and how Lee endured the boredom of spending every evening watching children's films I do not know. He was a star and this routine continued for about two years; it was not unusual for him to be up until two or three in the morning.

Once Mollie started taking melatonin, Lee could expect his film viewings to finish at around midnight. However, we had periods of months and months when she would refuse to take the melatonin, which would push her sleep back again.

Then, at the age of eight, we had a wonderful period where she would go to bed at about 11.00pm, take her melatonin and watch her iPad. Whoever took her to bed could expect to be an hour or more upstairs, due to her strategies to try and keep someone up there with her for as long as possible, but at least when that hour passed she did settle in her own bed and eventually go to sleep.

Then we went through a period of several months where she would be up all night and would often stay awake for 24 hours or more before crashing out. Because she was not in school, it really didn't matter and we could go with the flow. If she was awake all night she would remain in bed, usually in my bed with me, so we knew that she was safe. It was a bit like living with a shift worker but we had learned that there was nothing we could do to change the situation. The mere hint of a suggestion would push her to continue this routine even more avidly.

Eventually, under her own steam, she decided that she wanted to have the same sleeping pattern as everybody else. With no demands placed on her, it appeared that she found her own level in her own time and on her own terms. However, once she established a new and more typical sleep pattern it would only last for a few weeks or months before reverting to staying awake all night. This has now become a familiar sleep cycle for Mollie and rotates like clockwork.

We are hoping that within the next few years she will naturally decide to want to sleep in her own room again.

Transitions

This is another area of difficulty for Mollie. Leaving home, a swimming pool, a play area, school (even though she hated school), a stimulating shop or coming to the end of a day out can be problematic to say the least. Mollie appears to become stuck – unable to make the move from one situation to another.

She will use a variety of delaying tactics to stay where she is and to avoid the transition. When she finally makes the transition she can become extremely volatile. The slightest remark, or no remark at all, may prompt an outburst. It is important for us to remember first and foremost that a transition is in itself a demand. Also, Mollie appears to struggle with things coming to an end; she may prolong the event in order to prevent the low that she can experience at the end. We recently had to leave a pantomime before the end because watching right up until the end was too difficult for her.

If we are leaving the house, we give Mollie loads of notice and we tell her what time we need to be somewhere and then let her decide what time we need to leave. When she was younger she would need to carry an assortment of things with her whenever we went anywhere. These items are on assortment of Mollie's personal possessions, Blueberry Bear, a box of Barbie dolls, pens and colouring books. At the last minute she may decide that she just couldn't leave without taking a toy that we haven't seen for years. Eventually we would be able to leave, usually late, but stressful just wasn't the word for it.

I think that she needed all of those personal possessions to act as a comfort blanket and possibly to provide a link between one situation and the other. She now has an iPad, which provides a similar service. If she is watching an on-going film from the house to the car and from the car to our destination, the transitions appear to be much smoother.

If we are going somewhere that she will struggle to leave, we negotiate with her as to how long she may wish to stay at the venue. If we have agreed on a two-hour slot then we simply arrive two hours before closing. This greatly reduces the effort required in getting her to leave, because the instruction comes from a higher power and not from us. If the venue is closing she doesn't need to worry about missing out on any fun, as she would do if she was leaving while it was still open. She may still be very spiky and need handling with velvet gloves, and we do find it useful if we can offer her something to look forward to on the way home or when we return back, for example an ice cream, watching a film together or the promise of an hour's play. This sort of softens the blow and makes the end a little bit less of a straightforward cut off.

If we are going somewhere that doesn't have a closing time, such as the park, then, again, we offer her something to look forward to. We make leaving the park tempting by offering something nice that will follow and by being very patient and allowing her to leave in her own time with very gentle persuasion.

Whatever the transition, we always try to allow Mollie to feel that she is leaving at her own pace, in her own time and without the added pressure of being cajoled or feeling pushed to comply. She will do it eventually and, although it may seem longwinded and tedious, it will probably be quicker than going down the direct route, which may ultimately take longer and will certainly be far more emotionally draining.

Using a timer to count down to the end of an activity never worked with Mollie because she perceived this to be added pressure and a constant reminder that something good was coming to an end. However we have found a timer very useful for counting down to the start of a desired event.

Special events and holidays

Christmas, birthdays, Halloween, Easter and holidays, to name but a few, always cause a spike in behaviour in the build-up to the big day and induce huge amounts of anxiety. Mollie may be nervous about everything going to plan – the day must be perfect – which involves a lot of control.

Christmas and birthday's can induce anxiety because she may be worried about not receiving the exact gift that she has set her heart on. During the day of the event she may be on a complete high, which actually drives the demand avoidance to new levels, as well as the need to control. Towards the end of the day itself, she may experience difficulties coping with the fact that it will end. In the days following the event, her behaviour and control can be at a heightened level as she deals with the low of it all being over.

Imagine the stress a bride feels before her wedding day – all that planning over every tiny detail, panicking in case something goes wrong, the big build-up and the mounting tension turn many a woman into 'bridezilla'. When the day arrives, she is so busy making sure that everything is perfect and that everyone is doing what they should be that it almost seems as if it is over before it has begun. The day after the wedding can leave her feeling rather low and flat – the comedown after the high. Perhaps this is a good analogy of how Mollie may feel about events and holidays. So how can we lower the stress for her and make it more bearable for us?

We involve Mollie as much as possible in the planning so that she has a sense of control and ownership of an event. We also prepare for a spike in behaviour prior to the event. She may be more demanding of attention or have even more of a short fuse than normal; we try to remember that this is due to stress and anxiety.

If gifts are involved then we discuss what Mollie will be expecting with her, and if we are unable to meet the high expectations that she may have set, we negotiate. Mollie always knows, in advance, exactly what she will be receiving for her birthday and for Christmas.

When Mollie is excited or stressed, she needs one-on-one company to help her to stay calm. We ensure that for birthdays and Christmas she has as much one-to-one time as possible. These occasions tend to involve family social gatherings, so she seems to cope better if she has control of at least one person, which appears to alleviate the need to control the group. Adults work on a shift basis to provide cover so that the task becomes more manageable.

Some families may choose to have a very quiet and low-key occasion because this is what their child can cope with best. However, Mollie generally likes to have a big fuss and lots of family around – the scale of the event is really determined by your own child.

To avoid panic as the day is drawing to a close, perhaps due to the prospect of her expecting a low the next day, we try to spin things out. We may arrange something pleasant to look forward to for the following day. We try to make Boxing Day more appealing by making that the fun day that we explore all of the new gifts with complete one-on-one time. We may snuggle down under a duvet in the afternoon and watch a Christmas film with some tasty sweets and goodies.

Holidays are a very personal choice and ours have been greatly limited by Mollie's inability to cope with being in the car for any period of time. The iPad has helped in this area to some degree. All of our holidays are spent either in caravans or holiday homes because we need a home from home option so that we can comfortably stay in if she needs to have downtime and recharge. We may also decide to alter holidays to a few short breaks instead of a full week or fortnight.

The inability to wait, hyperactivity and boredom

Mollie appears to have huge difficulty with the concept of waiting for something. Whether it is waiting for me to fetch her a drink or respond to her demands, to receive a gift, for me to finish a meal or for a doctor's appointment in a waiting room, everything has to be instantaneous. I think that this may be a mixture of hyperactivity, boredom and a fear that if it isn't done straight away it won't get done at all. Waiting is, after all, a period of uncertainty.

If Mollie is excitedly waiting for the someone's arrival or for something fun to start then a timer is a useful way to help her cope with managing time. It can help to reduce the endless questioning of, 'How long now?' because she has something tangible to see.

If Mollie wants me, she wants me NOW, and that's all there is too it. This is something that I now accept and seldom fight against. I may occasionally delay the instant response by saying that I am just doing x, y and z but that I will be free in ten minutes if that is okay with her. She may give me a stay of execution if I have asked nicely and we may use the kitchen timer to indicate when my allowance of time has run out. It is important that I always follow through with my promise and do whatever it is that she wanted as soon as the time is up.

If Mollie wants an item now, or to go somewhere now, then my first thought is can I realistically achieve this or can I achieve this by just juggling a few things around? If I can do it, I will, because even if it is costing me money or interrupting any plans that I may have had, it is far easier to satisfy her need than to try and fight it. However, as she grows older, we are working on trying to teach her that other people may need advance warning and why.

If I need to keep Mollie occupied for a meal or a doctor's appointment then I always go with a bag of tricks to try to keep her occupied. The iPad is the only one that works successfully and it is only since she had this in January 2013 that life really has become so much more manageable. iPad, headphones plus Netflix have been pure gold in our household. Because watching films and TV have become her obsessions, it means that she is truly engaged during times that she would have previously been bored. A bored Mollie is a very disruptive Mollie.

Mollie is very hyperactive and she does score highly on the 'Connors Questionnaire', indicating possible ADHD. It may be that PDA in itself is a sufficient diagnosis, but it doesn't do any harm to recognise the high levels of impulsive and hyperactive behaviours that she exhibits.

It really is just a case of keeping her as engaged as possible with lots of different activities. As Mollie has grown older, and especially when she developed obsessions and routines, her hyperactivity has appeared to settle down. In our case, Mollie seems to be able to settle better if she has multiple input at any one time. If she is settled down with a film, providing her with lots of things to simultaneously colour in really helps her to sit still.

Interrupting and sabotaging communications with other people

Mollie went through a rather long phase of trying to and succeeding in cutting me off from all other human contact. She was frightened of me leaving her or someone trying to steal me and couldn't cope with not being in control of those actions or with not being the centre of attention. She would constantly interrupt any communications with others, switch phones off at the wall and attack or shock visitors into leaving and she also wanted me to wear no makeup, not do my hair and wear horrible clothes so that I was not deemed attractive or nice to other people. In any other relationship this would, I am sure, be considered an abusive relationship and it certainly felt that way a lot of the time.

We tried to deal with this by giving her a period of time where it really was just me and her, with minimal interference from anyone else. I would secretly make phone calls from the loo or email people as an alternative to phoning. Visitors were only allowed via appointment and during such visits we would make sure that someone else was in the house to entertain Mollie or for her to be taken out. In short, I needed a babysitter to facilitate me being able to talk to anybody.

Eventually we tried to expose her to short amounts of time coping with someone talking to me. If my parents visited, we would negotiate five minutes for them to talk to me and we used a timer so that Mollie felt sure that I couldn't sneak any extra time on. This would be followed by 20 minutes spent playing with her. Mollie would be in charge of the times and we gradually built up from there. However, this was a phase that naturally reduced with age, especially when she was mixing less socially and became more interested in her obsessions. It is a feature that often pops back for a visit though, especially when she is excited or nervous or senses excitement or tension in others.

Personal hygiene

A big area of concern for us is the subject of personal hygiene, especially the brushing of teeth, for obvious reasons. It has not been uncommon for Mollie to go weeks without brushing her teeth, brushing her hair or bathing. This particular area is one that seems to provoke an intense amount of avoidance. There may be sensory issues at work here, and depression and low self-esteem as well as the obvious demand avoidance.

This is an area that we found particularly difficult with Mollie – her hair would be matted, greasy and tangled, her teeth extremely yellow with bleeding gums and her body odour was intense, to say the least. We found these areas even more difficult to tackle during periods of low self-esteem or intensified anxiety due to an impending event.

Sensory issues made hair brushing extremely painful and the taste of toothpaste burned her mouth. The issue with bathing seemed to be based on the demand avoidance and the concept that bathing was boring and a waste of her time.

We would make gentle attempts each day, and throughout the day, in the hope that perhaps just one of these may be successful. I found that bathing was more likely to be achieved if I gently suggested a bath at the beginning of the day when she had just woken up and was still in bed. At this time, she was often at her calmest and had not been distracted by the events of the day. Each morning I would simply say, 'Would you like me to run you a lovely bath this morning?' and she would duly refuse. But on the odd occasion she would say yes and eventually we were achieving about two baths a week. The success of this would depend on how she was feeling internally.

We used the same technique for hair brushing but I would have a larger window of opportunity than I had for bathing. I would perhaps offer to brush her hair several times a day but without putting pressure on her to comply. Successes were few and far between, but it gradually grew into an achievable daily target. This, again, ebbs and flows depending on how well she is coping emotionally.

Teeth brushing became much more successful when we switched to an electric toothbrush and toothpaste for sensitive teeth. The gentle and softer flavouring of the toothpaste seemed more acceptable to her very sensitive palate. As with bathing and hair brushing, the occasional success gradually grew into almost daily brushing.

Obsessions

Mollie can become obsessed with another person, a game, a TV series or the desire to purchase a certain item. The obsession and the need to satisfy it really do know no bounds. Denying Mollie access to her obsession can provoke an endless round of begging, pleading, insisting and bargaining.

It can go on for hours, if not days, and the constant drip, drip effect is like torture. Her reserves of willpower and the mantra of 'never give up' will far outweigh mine and I am more likely to crack before she does. When she feels that this tactic is not going to bring around the desired result, or if I am standing my ground and insisting that, for example, I can't afford to take her to America for a Minecraft conference, it is prudent to brace myself for the meltdown from hell. Standing my ground, even when I have to, never appears to stop the behaviour occurring. Each family will have different boundaries regarding obsessions and to what extent and for how long they will allow their child to follow any given obsession. As long as Mollie is not harming anybody, we really allow her to lead her obsessions, although we gently try to advice and guide from the sidelines.

We would try to facilitate social obsessions as long as the other child was happy to proceed and wanted to play with Mollie. Play dates were nothing short of a nightmare, so we did negotiate with Mollie that we could only have friends around if two adults were in the house: one to help Mollie with any difficulties and one to protect or remove the other child if Mollie became too controlling or aggressive. This did make play dates manageable, with two girls in particular, but these did eventually come to a halt as the other girls grew up and spread their wings.

When she became totally obsessed with the children in the street, we were powerless to do anything other than let it run its natural course. We would have to physically remove her from the street if she was aggressive to other children. As much as we wanted her to avoid going out to play and gave her lots of alternative things to do, she was obsessed with the street and the children in it. It was with great relief that she finally decided to avoid this particular obsession, which was also such a huge trigger for her meltdowns. We could not impose this on her; we had to grit our teeth and cope as well as we could until she reached the decision.

Within the home, we do not restrict anything that Mollie wants to do. She has complete control of what she does and when, with no limitations over screen time. We do have periods when she may be up all night due to a mix of needing to continue with her obsession and her need to avoid the demand of sleep. We just let her get on with it while simultaneously offering to do other things with her in order to tempt her away from her obsession even if it is for just a little while.

We have found that with this full control, she naturally seems to find her own level where a suitable mix of engagement in other activities as well as the pursuit of her interest is achieved. I think that the important factor here is not to give up on the gentle and repetitive process of offering alternatives to any given obsession.

The relentless acquisition of goods, toys, sweets and so on is a really difficult one to deal with, because the need for Mollie to acquire the object becomes obsessional and refusal can result in a full meltdown. Of course, we can't just spend, spend, spend, so we have tried to think of other ways of setting some limits over spending rather than a direct no and the resulting meltdown. We had some success with negotiating a monthly allowance that Mollie could have control over. Goalposts will, of course, be repeatedly moved and the amount would be renegotiated, for example, 'Please can I have the new Barbie this month and you can take it off next month's money?' and so on. There are no set boundaries with Mollie and we always need to be flexible and to think on our feet, but this does at least put some structure into place. I deliberately gave Mollie an amount that I could easily manage so that I had some flexibility for the times when she would negotiate for other items.

If she suddenly wants something that she has seen on TV, if I can afford it I buy it, rather than enduring the constant bombardment, which will stress me out. I fully understand that she can't go through life having everything that she wants, but for now I choose my battles carefully. There will be plenty of times that I simply cannot afford the object of her desire and so I save my reserves for these periods rather than facing a standoff and the stress that goes with it if the item is easily within my budget.

When something can't be purchased – for financial or practical reasons – then this is when we just have to go through the eye of the storm. I may try to explain to her that when I have the money I will purchase the item but that I don't have the money right now. This may buy me a few months within which to renegotiate or to hope that the obsession passes and is, I hope, replaced by a less expensive one.

If the item just isn't feasible – either now or in the future – then I may just explain the reasons that it cannot be purchased and remain firm until she eventually backs down. These times will invariably pop up, and are draining to say the least, which is why I don't sweat the small stuff but retain all of my energy for the things that I simply can't supply.

At the age of ten, Mollie is now showing signs of being able to regulate her need for stuff and to spend within agreed limits. Occasionally this may go haywire but, overall, the need to spend impulsively without any apparent concern for money or where it will come from is steadily improving.

As Mollie got older we started giving her all of her birthday and Christmas money, from relatives and so on, to manage herself. This means we do have a small reserve pot of money for those impulsive buys and Mollie has control over her own little wad of money and, I hope, will learn the value of budgeting within a set amount.

Telling lies, fantasising, stealing and practical jokes

Mollie has, at times, appeared to relish telling lies to get others into trouble, telling tales of fantasy with elaborate fabricated stories, stealing and hiding family items and engaging in practical jokes that others seldom find funny.

To others, it may appear that she is being cruel, insensitive and deliberately misleading, and the practical jokes can get out of hand and appear malicious. However, the truth is that she either does these things for entertainment value or to try and make herself seem more interesting and appealing to others. I think that it is really important to play down this aspect of Mollie and to see it for what it really is: a mischievous little rascal having fun by playing tricks and watching the drama unfold, purely for the purpose of entertainment without fully understanding how inappropriate or poorly timed her escapades may be.

This understanding will come with age and maturity and is something that can be addressed in the future.

Mollie has stolen and hidden money, jewellery, anti-wrinkle cream, cheque books, watches, keys and games controllers, to name but a few. This has mainly been done just for the fun of watching the aftermath or for the thrill of getting away with it. Occasionally she has removed an item as a punishment for a perceived wrong that she has endured. Her dad's brand new iPod was missing for several days before she proudly boasted that she had thrown it in the bin as a punishment for him shouting at her.

As a rule, we now try to see the funny side of such incidents rather than getting angry with her because she simply doesn't appear to understand, at an emotional level, the implications that her bit of fun or calculated revenge may have had on others. As with many areas of PDA, this is improving as she gets older. A couple of days ago she hid every car key in the house and lay in bed chuckling as she heard us frantically searching for the keys. I took it in good humour when the keys were located hidden in a greetings card box. I laughed as I told her that her dad had walked to work and her brother had received a late mark in school. I didn't laugh because I thought that it was funny, but it was a way of me conveying to Mollie how disruptive that prank had been in an unthreatening manner. That night she apologised to her brother and dad for the trouble that it had caused.

When it comes to her stories and tales of fantasy, we just go with the flow rather than correcting her. Often it is merely a ploy to try and build up her own self-esteem by making herself appear more interesting and appealing to others. She just wants us to play along and as long as it isn't hurting anyone else then we really don't see the harm in it. If she is deceiving another child then we may discreetly tell the other child and explain that it is part of her condition.

Many of her tales are so far-fetched that even another child may have difficulty believing her, which can make Mollie extremely agitated. In such situations we just try and distract her or move on to a different topic. Some of the stories are so funny and we truly wonder how she thinks them up – for us this is one of the more endearing features of her PDA and isn't something that we feel we need to stamp out and is something that we can secretly smile about.

Mollie sometimes tries to get her brother in to trouble by telling tales about things that he has done; I wonder if these are lies or her perceived reality of the situation. She can demand that he is scolded for his crime and will not relent until this is done. My son and I have a special code during such times and so he is told off, receives the wink and gracefully plays the game. Mollie is happy, he is happy and the house is calm.

Swearing

Mollie swears like a trooper and the really offensive language began when she was about eight years old. Her language had been very cheeky prior to this period but was limited by her small vocabulary of swear words. Sadly this is no longer the case and her repertoire has grown.

The 'F word' is a particular favourite of hers usually accompanied by the middle finger gesture. Mollie was so volatile and violent during the ages of four and nine that swearing was, to be honest, the least of my problems. Being sworn at was preferable to dodging a flying missile or being repeatedly kicked. We decided to completely ignore the swearing and, to be fair, she did seem to be able to moderate her use of swear words – they would generally only tumble out during periods of extreme anger and within the home.

If we reacted to a swear word, then her anger, anxiety or upset would be cranked up to the next level. Ignoring it meant that everything would settle down more quickly, and experience had taught me that trying to stamp out any undesirable behaviour simply intensified it.

If Mollie swore in the street in front of younger children then that was not acceptable and she would be moved indoors. However, if the only audience were family members then we turned a blind eye and would often not even acknowledge it. Now that Mollie is calmer and living in a more suitable environment, the swearing has, for the most part, declined.

Because she is now calmer and less volatile, when Mollie does swear I can gently say that I wished she wouldn't because I really don't like to hear that kind of language. This gentler way of addressing the issue means that I can voice my opinion without it getting her back up. I hope that she may decide of her own accord that if swearing produces no reaction, she will continue to reduce the use of it.

Mess, mess and more mess

Wherever Mollie goes she tends to leave a trail of destruction in her wake. I cannot even begin to project accurately the vast amount of time I have to spend on a daily basis simply keeping on top of the continual mountains of mess that she creates. When she plays, everything has to be on a grand scale and the room that she is playing in is turned into a movie set.

The kitchen is quickly turned into a hairdressing salon with tons of beautifying products, dolls, doll makeover heads, teddy bears and so on. Hair is sprayed and cut while makeup flies around being dropped on the floor and slapped onto dolls' faces. Then it can be my turn for a makeover, and I often end up looking like a zombie with a ten-combination pigtail affair for a hairdo.

While I try and tidy up the huge mess in the kitchen, she will turbocharge into the hallway and empty the cupboard under the stairs. Several hundred pairs of shoes will now be lying all over the hallway, complete with a few bags. Meanwhile, Mollie can be found under the stairs along with a small table from the lounge, a rug and a lamp, as happy as anything in her new den.

Five minutes later and the den will lose its novelty value. I'll still be trying to tidy up the kitchen, getting stressed in the knowledge that I now have all the shoes to sort out and watching in horror as she darts into the conservatory.

Oh no, is that glitter I can see?! She's making a glitter potion, the glitter gets everywhere and still she hasn't finished. Oh no, the paints and plaster of Paris are coming out. She needs me to find the moulds and make the mixture up. It doesn't matter that I am now drowning in mess and that my home looks like an episode of *Can't Stop, Won't Stop: Hoarding*. She can't wait – it has to be done now!

In addition to the play mess that she creates, Mollie is 'positively allergic' to any suggestion of tidying up – plates and cups are left where she has eaten, toilets are left un-flushed, wrappers and cartons are discarded on floors and desks, and this is just the tip of the iceberg.

I have accepted my fate in life as that of a carer and unpaid skivvy. Pushing the demand for tidiness just leads us down a rocky road to nowhere and it is ultimately far quicker to do it myself. I just class the constant mess and the continual tidying up as part of my job as Mollie's mum and carer.

That doesn't mean to say that I don't gently, and with careful timing, strive for small improvements. On an odd day a toy may be tidied away or a plate may appear at the side of the sink instead of being left in the lounge. All I know is that the harder I push, the less success I have and the gentler and softer I make suggestions, the more likelihood I have of small improvements.

Limited repertoire of food

I have experienced this issue with both of my children. I found it extremely worrying when they would only eat the same food day after day, and anything other than a specific type of food would actually make them gag. The factors that appeared to underpin this problem were the taste, smell, look and texture of the food, due to sensory issues, in conjunction with the need for repetition.

At one stage, other than cereal, Jake would only eat potato smiley faces, southern fried chicken pieces and beans. Any attempts to encourage him to eat different foods simply caused undue stress for both of us and never resulted in him eating anything different or broadening his repertoire. I was much more relaxed when Mollie exhibited the same difficulties because I had already experienced this with my son.

I simply fed them both the food that they would eat, even if it was the same food day in and day out and even if it wasn't particularly healthy. The way I looked at the situation was that I would rather have a full and satisfied child fed on a diet of chicken nuggets and smiley faces than a stressed and hungry child eating nothing due to food refusal. I took the attitude that I needed to reduce any stress that my children associated with food.

I gradually tried to tempt, encourage and offer them different food choices by preparing them a tiny portion of whatever Lee and I were having for our evening meal, such as cottage pie. Then I would serve them their usual evening meal with a small side portion of cottage pie for them to try if they wanted to.

This reduced the pressure associated with food. They had the chance to try new foods safe in the knowledge that they still had a meal of their usual food. If the side dish was approved it would be introduced as a new regular meal within their diet.

This area has improved as my children have got older and they both now enjoy a varied diet. However, if we are trying something new I still use the side portion method to introduce it, so there is no stress or pressure associated with the new food. As my children have matured they have also developed a desire to try new things and they appear to be less afraid of food.

My son now eats practically anything and everything that is edible while also keeping to a healthy diet. Mollie is a little bit more complex because food is consumed for comfort as well as when she is hungry. Her repertoire of food has greatly improved but we do have difficulty controlling the amount of food that she craves on a daily basis. Fortunately she has always been a great lover of fruit, so we try to replace unhealthy snacks with fruit whenever we can.

Sexualised behaviour
Some children with PDA, including Mollie, appear to be born with an instinctive and natural amount of sexual

awareness that can be extremely disconcerting to both their families and others. At a very young age some individuals may display sexualised and provocative behaviour that you would not expect to see in a typically developing child of a similar age. This is information that I have gleaned from my personal experience with Mollie and through sharing experiences with other parents. However, it is not, as far as I am aware, currently thought to be a prolific or notable feature of PDA.

This behaviour may wrongly, but understandably, lead other people involved with the child to assume that the child may be, or has been, a victim of sexual abuse. This can lead to families having to endure investigations by social services. It is vitally important for any concerns regarding a child to be taken seriously, but I also think that it is important for services to be aware that this seems to be a behaviour displayed by some children with PDA and the underlying cause is not automatically going to be abuse.

Mollie had not been abused or exposed to age-inappropriate material when she first started to display this concerning behaviour. Therefore, I can only assume that this early sexualised awareness is instinctive, due to nature alone and not influenced by nurture.

The only external force that influenced one particular behaviour from Mollie was Power Rangers, believe it or not. She witnessed a boy and a girl engaging in a kiss at the end of one of the shows. She then went on a spree of trying to kiss, with an open mouth – that is, a grown up kiss, everyone and anyone.

I have a feeling that she was only about three or four at the time. I tried to explain to her that this type of kiss wasn't suitable between a child and an adult or a family member. I discussed with her how this type of kiss was only to be engaged in when she was much older and with her chosen partner at that time. Here is, I think, a clear case of Mollie's deep confusion and lack of intuitively understanding correct behaviours or when and where certain behaviours should take place.

According to my own experience and other parental descriptions, behaviours exhibited by some children with PDA can include removing their clothes, flashing their genitalia, making provocative poses and touching others inappropriately.

It would now appear, with Mollie's insight, that some of her behaviours were not actually intended to be sexual as such – she simply delighted in the reactions that this behaviour provoked in others, especially if it achieved the desired result of shocking somebody out of the house.

This type of behaviour calmed down between the ages of about seven and nine and it doesn't occur at all now. She can still be inappropriate but this is now expressed verbally rather than by her actions.

When Mollie attended her third school placement she was, due to the lack of a suitable peer group, placed with boys who were several years older than her. Unfortunately they gave Mollie a rather rapid and crude education on all things sexual. So she then had the actual facts to accompany her already overdeveloped natural awareness. I am a very liberal and open-minded individual, who is not easily embarrassed, but even I was totally shocked by what she would openly blurt out at home as a result of her newly acquired information.

With puberty now in full swing, even though she is only ten years old, these sexual feelings and the urge to explore this area could take on a whole new level. It is natural for any individual to want to explore such urges and to learn about sex, but it was and still is vitally important to us that Mollie is not overexposed to inappropriate material.

A child may typically learn slowly and gradually, often through other children, and then go on to develop crushes and budding, fledgling relationships. These relationships can then move slowly forward from handholding to kissing and to petting as children mature into teenagers and young adults.

This avenue is not currently open to Mollie, so we attempted to safeguard her in an area that any enquiring mind may choose to explore: the internet. I felt that she may be sexually vulnerable, so I needed to feel safe in the knowledge that she wasn't being exposed to really unacceptable images that she may then assume are normal. This could leave her very vulnerable to being easily taken advantage of by unscrupulous individuals as she grows older.

Even with safety settings activated on her iPad, we discovered that it was still possible to access inappropriate material. So, on the advice of a fellow parent, we adjusted the setting on our router so that no adult material could be accessed. Fortunately, the internet available at home is now a safe area to explore. I do understand that it is totally natural for Mollie to want to explore such topics, so I have told her to feel free to ask me anything that she wants to know. Mollie's sexual vulnerability coupled with her appearing to have few inhibitions is an area over which we shall remain constantly vigilant.

External influences

Despite our very best efforts within the home and the family to enthusiastically embrace and implement the strategies, we did sometimes feel as if we were completely swimming against the tide when they were not duplicated by the outside world.

In short, all of our hard work and the calmness that we were providing for Mollie were rapidly undone unless the same understanding and ethos were also adopted by others. Of course, it was not realistic to expect the whole world to suddenly adapt to Mollie, but during certain periods she was unable to adapt or to cope with them either. We had reached stalemate!

The two biggest external influences that hindered Mollie's recovery and kept her in a perpetual state of self-loathing and high anxiety were the repeated attempts, by her, to play in the street with the neighbours' children and the repeated attempts at formal education.

Even though her schools did adopt PDA strategies, she just couldn't cope with the pressure of daily exposure to the outside world.

When it came to playing with other children we tried to advise Mollie that choosing to do so was only bringing her negative experiences. Playing in the street was akin to being let loose and unsupervised in a playground and as she grew older she seemed to be able to cope with it less and less.

Socialising was causing mammoth and multiple meltdowns on a daily basis and was not producing anything positive for Mollie other than crushing her already fragile self-esteem. The stress on the family was untenable and, as her mother, I also had to consider the effect that Mollie was having on other children. Eventually Mollie made the sensible choice to stop playing in the street.

Even though Mollie has been extremely lucky with our LEA, and has been given all the support that she could possibly have, she still couldn't cope with school attendance. The process of trying to hold it together and cope with social interaction, and the bombardment of sensory stimuli outside of the family on a daily basis, was not feasible for her.

Despite all our strategies, understanding and support, we were still struggling with Mollie who was, at that time, nine years old. The huge meltdowns had diminished at home but whenever she was reintroduced to a new school the meltdowns and high anxiety would reappear and the full effects of her struggle would be absorbed and felt at home. It was only when we decided to completely remove formal education from Mollie's life that our real journey and the healing process truly began. Without any external influences we could really start to lay the foundations for the future and gradually rebuild our shattered and broken daughter.

Applying the basic foundation strategies, and having awareness and strategies for the other areas of difficulty for Mollie, had not made our daughter any less complex or challenging but they had reduced her anxiety, which had in turn almost completely eliminated the meltdowns and the very extreme behaviour. It was important for us to remember that successful strategies appeared to have a certain shelf life. We would often need to chop, change and rotate them.

I think a common theme that runs through how we manage Mollie can be broken down into a simple format:

- Picking my battles – what is important and what isn't?

- Is this behaviour or action going to hurt either Mollie or someone else?

- Is it going to be quicker, easier and less stressful to just go with the flow rather than resist and stand my ground?

- Can I work on this issue in a more productive and gentler manner over a gradual period of time rather than here and now?

- Progress and improvements take time and patience – there is no quick fix.

- The lower the demands, the lower the anxiety and the fewer the meltdowns. Only when Mollie is at her calmest can we reasonably expect any progress or compliance with demands.

The purpose of applying these strategies and trying to understand the behaviour is not to cure PDA, because our child and PDA are inextricably linked. The personality traits and behaviours of PDA are part of what makes our child who she is. It is not our quest to eradicate the true essence of our child but to provide her with the optimum environment to be the best that she can be. It took us several years to undo the damage that years of incorrect behaviour strategies coupled with too much social exposure had caused. PDA is not for the faint-hearted and there is no quick fix.

13

Getting School Right

There is informative and helpful information about the most appropriate educational provision for children with PDA in the book *Understanding Pathological Demand Avoidance in Children* (Christie *et al.* 2011). Some children's PDA seems to affect them at home more than in school. These children may need relatively little to accommodate their needs in the school setting. For most though, considerable adaptation is needed to reduce their anxiety and enable them to access learning and wider social opportunities. The sorts of features that are usually characteristic of an appropriate educational provision include an understanding of PDA and the strategies that are likely to be helpful, additional support in the classroom, a flexible attitude and a personalised approach and curriculum, together with a willingness to work openly with the family. However, because of our decision not to pursue a formal education for Mollie, this chapter shall mainly focus on an alternative option to formal schooling.

The path that we ultimately took for Mollie's education was created by personal choice and is not one that is necessarily recommended by the professionals involved in

PDA. However, it is the one that has, so far, proved the most successful for Mollie.

Mollie's second school placement offered her excellent provision; I truly believe that there is nothing more that they could have done in order to ensure success. The fact that this placement failed serves as a testament to Mollie's complexities and is not a reflection on anything that the school did wrong.

Mollie had a full-time 2:1 staffing ratio, however I feel that this may have overwhelmed her and she may have coped better with a 1:1 staffing ratio split between two staff members, which would also have reduced the stress on staff. Unfortunately this couldn't be done, because Mollie's explosive outbursts meant that two people would always need to be on hand in case they needed to physically restrain her.

Mollie's special needs teacher initially made home visits and educated herself on PDA in order to build a relationship with Mollie prior to her beginning school. She then introduced Mollie to the lady who would be her teaching assistant (TA) and they continued with home visits. Both the special needs teacher and the TA adopted the same understanding, strategies and means of communicating with Mollie as illustrated in the previous chapters.

The home visits were gradually phased out and replaced with a series of short visits to the school. The length and frequency of these visits was built up at Mollie's pace. During this time Mollie was introduced to her second TA, and the special needs teacher gradually withdrew. This allowed the two TAs who would be providing Mollie with her 2:1 staffing ratio to build and strengthen relationships.

Mollie was given her own room that she could decorate and design to her own tastes, and she was not expected to wear a school uniform. She was allowed to have personal items and toys from home in her room to provide comfort.

She was given the choice of attending lessons or staying in her own room and doing activities of her choice with her TA. She would often choose the classroom over her own room, especially if the itinerary in the classroom was kinetic learning, for example science experiments, arts and crafts or rehearsing for plays.

The school actively tried to integrate Mollie with other children so that she had positive peer interaction and she could invite children to come and play in her room at break times and for golden time. The school day was completely child led and dictated by Mollie.

Any arising difficulties were discussed with us and a combined effort was made to smooth over any rough edges. The priority for the school, and for us, was simply for Mollie to attend school and to enjoy being there. All of the parties concerned agreed that a formal education was secondary to her social education. It may be possible to negotiate with children who are more amenable to demands regarding times to learn and times to play.

With the correct support, many children do manage to continue to attend school on a full-time basis. Unfortunately for Mollie, no amount of support could suppress the huge anxiety that this type of daily social exposure was causing her.

Even with all of this support and the faultless management by staff, the meltdowns in school began to grow and intensify, leading to the return of school refusal. Following the breakdown of her second school placement Mollie attended her third school placement which was an ASD specialised school. However, within a few months, we were again experiencing school refusal. It was during this period that we finally addressed the fact that the pursuit of a school that Mollie could cope with was no longer a realistic option. Christie *et al.* (2011) explain that for some children home education does become the last viable option: 'It is sometimes a necessity for some parents whose children may be too anxious to even leave the house or be recurrent school refusers' (Christie *et al.* 2011, p.137).

We finally officially removed Mollie from formal education when she was nine years old. This has been the most important decision that we have made and has been the single most defining decision in helping us to turn Mollie around.

Home-schooling

This is a deeply personal decision, because home-schooling just isn't a viable option for many families. Parents may feel strongly that they want their child to receive a formal education, they may be concerned that having their child at home all day could further undermine an already fragile relationship or there may be financial reasons that just make this decision unfeasible. There are no right or wrong answers when it comes to home-schooling; it really is up to each individual family to do what is right for them.

Alternatively many parents may feel that they have no choice but to home educate due the needs of their child not being met by their Local Authority. This may not be a positive or a desirable outcome for many families, although it is noted that this may be the best option for some individuals with PDA as discussed by Christie *et al.* (2011):

> It may feel like a last resort after a string of failed placements, creating financial hardship and feelings of resentment towards an education system that has failed them and their child. This 'last resort' option is

not ideal, as it may not be beneficial for either parent, child or their relationship. For some parents, though, it is a positive choice to home educate, and it may, in fact, be the best option for them. (Christie *et al.* 2011, pp.136–137)

Following a disastrous attempt to actually teach Mollie at home, which led to the complete withdrawal of Mollie from me (which shall be discussed in the next chapter), I studied the philosophy of 'unschooling'. While this method of learning may not be ideal for many children, it was a lifesaver for me.

I won't go into detail about the legalities here, because there is plenty of information available on the internet for those who wish to know their full legal rights within this area. What I will say is that as the law currently stands in England (July 2014) parents are legally entitled to home educate their children following an autonomous approach; another term used for this method of home education is 'unschooling'.

Laws and legislation may be different in other countries and subject to change, therefore it is advisable to investigate the legal position in your area if home-schooling is something that you are considering. There are an array of websites and Facebook groups that offer up-to-the-minute, free, legal advice, support and information.

It is currently not a legal requirement for children to go to school, but it is a legal requirement that all children should receive an education. If you decide to home-school your child, you simply need to write to the school declaring your intention to 'educate otherwise' from (state the date that you hope to begin) and request that the school removes your child's name from the school register.

If your child is attending a specialised placement then you need to write to the LEA declaring your intention to 'educate otherwise' and request its permission for the school to remove your child's name from the school register. Your LEA should not refuse permission unless it has very good reasons. This is simply a precaution to ensure that the special needs of potentially vulnerable children are being met.

It is a criminal offence, and you can be penalised or prosecuted, if your child is registered with a school and you simply stop sending him/her. Whether you are intending to home-school or your child is school refusing, always keep the school informed of your situation.

Once you are home-schooling, you are free to do so in any way that you please. There are no laws stipulating a curriculum that must be followed, lessons that must be taught, tests that must be taken or work that must be recorded.

As long as your child has access to you and to learning materials, for example pencils, pens, paper, age-appropriate reading material, arts and crafts and computers and so on, and you are meeting any special needs requirements, then you are fulfilling your legal obligation as required by current legislation.

Requirements of the law as stated in Part 2 point 2.3 of 'Elective Home Education: Guidelines for Local Authorities' states that the responsibility for a child's education rests with his or her parents. An 'efficient' and 'suitable' education is not defined in the Education Act 1996 but 'efficient' has been broadly described in case law as an education that 'achieves that which it sets out to achieve', and a 'suitable' education is one that:

> Primarily equips a child for life within the community of which he is a member, rather than the way of life in the country as a whole, as long as it does not foreclose the child's options in later years to adopt some other

form of life if he wishes to do so. (Mr Justice Woolf in the case of *R v Secretary of State for Education and Science* [1985] ex parte Talmud Torah Machzikei Hadass School Trust, cited in Department for Children, School and Families 2007, 2013)

The philosophy of unschooling

Prior to attending school, many children have already naturally learnt how to walk, talk and play, among many other skills. These skills have not necessarily being taught to the child but have been learnt at their own pace simply through living and exploring their immediate environment. It is believed that if children are left to their own devices, they will naturally learn through play and by following their own interests (Thomas and Pattison 2009).

Parents are instrumental in ensuring that they facilitate their child being able to learn through play and following their interests, but it is not their role to instigate learning or the direction that any given interest should take. Of course, this doesn't mean that parents should sit sipping a can of beer and watching daytime TV and just leave their kids to get on with it. What it does mean is that parents can allow their child to follow his/her own interests, provide their child with the appropriate materials in order to do so (paper, pens, computer equipment, literature and so on), be available to assist their child with various projects and be an active and interested participant in their child's daily living.

I joined a few unschooling Facebook groups, read applicable literature and researched the topic. I was surprised to find that many children thrive on this philosophy of learning, growing into very well adjusted and confident young adults. When they reach a certain age, they often have a clear direction of which path in life they wish to explore and many choose to go to college and then on to university to study their chosen area of interest:

> Compared to the careful way in which the curriculum is presented in school, the chaotic nature of input from everyday cultural knowledge and the individual led interests of children themselves, seem like a chancy combination. It nevertheless does seem that the informal curriculum is as good a preparation as any for moving into formal education. Children entered the formal system, either by going to school, college or university or by taking up home-based formal courses such as correspondence courses at around the GCSE (year 11) level or later. Whenever this stage arrived for them personally, it seems that the young people themselves were able to decide on their own terms what and how they wanted to study and had both sufficient subject knowledge and study and personal skills to make the transition with apparent ease. (Thomas and Pattison 2009, p.47)

For our family, this was the only option available, because any type of structured teaching just caused Mollie to avoid me even more and she became harder to reach on all levels. I also have to admit that all of my life skills and skills in the workplace did not come from what I had learned at school, most of which I have forgotten, but came, instead, from hands-on experience and from learning as I went along. The same can be said for my husband, who for most of his school experience was being caned or he was skipping school altogether. He developed an interest in electrics after he had left school, chose to study it at college and now runs his own business designing and building bespoke kilns for glass artists.

I suppose what I am trying to convey is that a formal education is, for some, not the be all and end all. My opinion is that specific topics or areas of education can be learnt at any time during your life, as and when it may be necessary and dependent on individual circumstances. It isn't mandatory that these specific areas must be learnt between the ages of 4 and 16; education is a process that continues throughout life. I was beginning to see the possible merits of unschooling and why many families choose to take this option regardless of whether their child has any special education needs.

That being said, I am not against formal education; my son still attends mainstream school and he is doing well. I think that being at home all day would have been a disaster for him, because he has learnt from and thrived on the accompanying social interaction and friendships that school provides. However, for Mollie, I was forced to think more outside the box as far as her education was concerned. We needed to implement a very individual pathway in order to meet her needs at that time. As they say, 'one size does not fit all', so we chose two alternative paths of education for our children based on their specific needs at that time.

For many parents, a child's academic progress may be of less importance, during certain periods, than their social development and emotional well-being. By following a philosophy of unschooling, we have been able to focus solely on this area and we are beginning to see the fruits of our labour. In the years to come, it may even be possible for Mollie to consider returning to formal education, but that shall depend entirely upon her progress. I am hopeful that with the correct support and guidance now, she may at some point be able to attempt a college course in her area of interest.

Following on from this is the proposal that I made to the LEA outlining the home education that I would be providing for Mollie.

MOLLIE'S PROPOSED STATEMENT

Mollie's diagnosis at the age of six was 'Asperger's', 'sensory processing disorder' and 'major visual perceptual problems' consistent with those described as 'Irlen syndrome'. At the age of seven, Mollie was diagnosed with PDA by Phil Christie at the Elizabeth Newson Centre. Pathological Demand Avoidance syndrome is described in her diagnostic report from the Elizabeth Newson Centre as an autism spectrum disorder and this diagnosis overrides her diagnosis of Asperger's syndrome. It was the opinion of the Elizabeth Newson Centre that Mollie's profile of ASD most closely fitted that of PDA and not that of Asperger's syndrome.

Description of the home education provision provided by me for the first four months of home-schooling

From the moment that I finally decided to home-school Mollie, I adopted an approach of trying to follow the national curriculum. I have tried to teach Mollie in a creative and non-pressured manner, allowing for her to engage as and when she wanted. We had an encouraging start and we managed to learn a substantial amount given that she appeared to spend most of her time actively avoiding joining in.

I do feel that she learned and gained a lot from the dinosaur topic, however I feel that everything that we have done since then has been rather pointless and that she has not absorbed any information.

I have gone to great lengths to research topics, think of lots of different ways of presenting the information and to be creative and flexible. Unfortunately, the result has been complete withdrawal and we now find ourselves in a position where nothing productive is currently being achieved, which is why I have had to look at alternative methods.

As well as withdrawing, she also appears depressed and her general interaction skills within the family setting have become non-existent.

The type of approach that I initially adopted and the work that we did can be seen in the books, folders and photographic evidence that I have presented.

Objectives for Mollie's education at home and for the future

- To try to halt the rapid deterioration in Mollie's emotional well-being.

- For Mollie to be happy and at peace with herself and who she is.

- For Mollie to develop an understanding of her condition and to be accepting of it.

- To try to encourage a much improved level of personal hygiene.

- To try to encourage Mollie to eat healthier food and to engage in more exercise.

- To try to enable Mollie to feel more comfortable leaving the house and deriving enjoyment from suitable activities outside of the home.

- To follow Mollie's lead in areas that she shows an interest in and to enable her to explore these interests to whatever level she desires.

- To protect Mollie from negative comments from others, which only serve to lower self-esteem.

- To allow Mollie to learn naturally from her environment by adopting an autonomous approach.

- Mollie can tell the time, read (within the limits of her dyslexia), do basic maths (manage her money in a shop), operate a computer, operate her iPad, operate the TV and DVD player, play a variety of computer games and make her own breakfast and drinks, amongst other things. All of these skills have been acquired through life rather than being specifically taught. Of course, whilst she has the ability to do these things, her PDA will often not allow her to.

Provision to meet needs and objectives for the future

- Mollie has access to a large play area and a large garden. Her play area is 23 foot by 13 foot and is extremely well stocked with toys, arts and crafts materials, a large TV, Xbox 360, Xbox Kinect , a computer and a printer.

- Either myself or Lee will be available to play with Mollie at virtually all times throughout the day, with exception to when other duties need to be performed, for example housework, cooking, cleaning and so on.

- We have recently purchased Mollie two pairs of new glasses; one pair is to help her deal with her over-sensitivity to sunlight and the other pair has tinted red lenses, which dramatically reduce the effects of Irlen syndrome.

- We also have access to educational resources should Mollie want to explore these further: books, the internet, educational games on her iPad, DVDs and so on.

- We shall be aiming to give Mollie a full educational day out once a month, for example the zoo, a museum, a theme park and so on, depending on the weather, time of year and her willingness to take part.

- We shall also be aiming to increase the amount of short outings that Mollie currently accesses, for example to the cinema. Again, this also depends on Mollie's anxiety levels and whether she is able to attend or not.

- To increase the opportunities for Mollie to access peers but to limit this to short, bite-sized chunks rather than extended periods of time, to protect her from this developing into a negative experience, whilst still offering her the chance to mix with other children.

- Mollie will have access to reading material in the form of comics and downloaded books for her to read should she choose to do so. She avoids reading due to the dyslexic nature of her Irlen syndrome, however she does read when it is not enforced, for example computer games, road signs, baking instructions etc. This material will be suitable for her age and ability; it must be remembered that although Mollie is very bright, her reading is below where it should be due to the dyslexic nature of her 'major visual perception difficulties'. Words move, vibrate, blur and float around on the page. This could, of course, be completely remedied by Mollie wearing her 'orthoscopic lenses', which she refuses to do, as this is a demand.

- Mollie has constant access to a computer to play her favourite games. This has been the greatest resource to date from the point of view of improving literacy skills. Games such as Minecraft can be very educational.

- Due to Mollie's PDA, it is impossible to have a structured setting or to teach in either a formal or a non-formal way. This child will avoid all perceived demands, and on a bad day even answering a question will be avoided due to the associated demand. Therefore, any learning has to be child led in order for progress to be made. Following an autonomous approach to learning is catering specifically for

Mollie's special education needs in a way that structured or traditional learning just can't.

- Mollie enjoys play sessions with her personal assistant, with whom she has a very strong relationship. This provides her with the opportunity to increase her social skills in a play-based environment.

- We feel that the objectives of what we would like to achieve with Mollie will be best met by the philosophy of unschooling and that this method will achieve the optimum results for Mollie.

- From an emotional point of view, Lee and I are available for Mollie day or night to discuss or help her with any issues that she may have. Again, this needs to be child led; asking for Mollie to divulge information regarding her feelings simply leads to a confrontation because this is viewed as a demand.

I believe that the provision outlined above will meet the requirements of the law as stated in Part 2 point 2.3 of the Elective Home Education Guidelines For Local Authorities.

Due to Mollie's special needs, we have to be realistic in the fact that her community may be limited to that of her close family. However we shall be endeavouring to expand Mollie's community to also include a close circle of friends outside of the family circle with whom she feels comfortable.

Mollie is now ten-and-a-half years old and has now been home-schooled for a period of just over one year. We are making steady progress in meeting the objectives of this proposed statement.

With the removal of formal teaching, we have been able to allow her to learn naturally while simultaneously repairing her damaged self-esteem and crushed confidence, which I shall discuss in the next chapter.

Mollie spends a lot of time playing on her computer while watching TV shows, films, YouTube videos on her iPad and so on. During other periods she may play Lego or colour in or engage in arts and crafts while she has the white noise of her iPad on in the background. She appears to require multiple inputs to facilitate concentration.

Many of the games she plays are educational and mentally stimulating. Mollie also researches many of her interests and searches for instructions on how to do things on the computer. Her reading and writing has improved tenfold by simply learning naturally and having to navigate and search for information. The hands-on approach and visual learning that demonstration videos on YouTube offer her have proved to be a much more relaxing and successful method of her learning how to do new things.

Mollie loves making films on her iPad to which she adds music, special effects and credits. Allowing her simply to do her own thing and by using all of the strategies outlined in the next chapter, has resulted in her steadily coming out of her withdrawal and she now actively seeks more social interaction within the family and with peers.

She enjoys playing board games, like Monopoly, which promote reading, maths and managing her money. Of course she cheats and has to win but, with the lower level of anxiety that she now experiences within the home, simply playing the game has become a viable option.

Following a period of acute social exposure anxiety (which shall be discussed in the next chapter), we eventually made extremely tentative steps outside of the home. A short period on medication greatly assisted us in this area but we had to discontinue it due to the side effects. Mollie is, however, now prescribed fluoxetine, which has lowered her general anxiety levels, although it does nothing for her PDA.

With lower anxiety she is enjoying occasional trips out when she feels she can cope with the outside world. These are steadily growing in frequency, but we still have periods when she is unable to go out at all. She continues to enjoy her play dates with Ann and she has been steadily venturing outside and making friends with other children in her street, which we shall discuss more in the next few chapters.

Personal hygiene has vastly improved and she appears to accept this with far less reluctance than previously, although this can ebb and flow depending on a variety of other influencing factors at any given time.

She is beginning to understand herself and her condition much more, and she is more open to discussing how she feels. Self-awareness has, for us, been such a huge step in the right direction. I have always been open with her – first with regard to her Asperger's diagnosis and second with her PDA diagnosis.

The more I learn and understand about PDA, the more open our lines of communication have become. If I talk her language and describe to her how I feel that she may understand or interpret the world, this does appear to give her a few light-bulb moments of her own, such as: 'Ah, so I'm not completely on my own, other people do see and interpret the world in the same way as me', 'Mum does understand me and she can help me understand why I behave and react in the way that I do', 'Oh so that's why life can be so tough it's because other people don't understand me because they are wired differently to me' and so on.

In conclusion, I think that it is fair to say that the removal of school was instrumental and an absolute necessity in order for us to move forward in a positive direction with Mollie. While she was continuing to live in a state of permanent anxiety of either attending school or being at home, due to school refusal, but waiting with trepidation for a new school placement to start, she was never calm or at peace. However, I would not rule out a return to formal education if it is an area that Mollie ever feels able to attempt again. I imagine that this is more likely to be a possibility when she approaches college age.

14

PDA Plus

Some children with PDA become more reclusive as they get older. It would be natural to assume that Mollie's inability to leave the home was purely down to the demands associated with it; however, I feel that it is important to recognise that some children may develop PDA Plus. This is a term coined by a very knowledgeable and experienced friend of mine named Neville Starnes.

Children who have PDA coupled with insufficient support and understanding and incorrect handling may go on to develop other psychological issues that may need to be looked at and managed alongside their central condition. Anxieties associated with being misunderstood, years of people around them using the incorrect strategies, high levels of anxiety-provoking social exposure and the possibility of public meltdowns, in my opinion, caused low self-esteem, exacerbated Mollie's levels of anxiety outside the home and led to periods of depression.

I suppose that a good analogy would be to imagine an individual with alopecia. The hair loss is the central difficulty but this in itself may then cause many more mental health issues. The individual may suffer a confidence crisis and feel unattractive to others and self-conscious in public because they may feel that others stare at them. This could lead to depression and a lack of self-esteem, and they may feel more comfortable withdrawing from many social occasions or experiences. The central feature of alopecia will always be there, but the individual may benefit hugely from having support and help with dealing with the other mental health issues that are a direct result of the central difficulty, in conjunction with support in helping them to accept the central difficulty.

Mollie was about six years old when she first started to avoid going out. Refusal to leave the home really began with school refusal and it gradually permeated all aspects of her social life. She would refuse to go to shops, parks and anywhere else that she didn't want to go to, due to a combination of increasingly high levels of anxiety combined with the issue of being more and more reluctant to go anywhere that she didn't feel personally benefited her. I didn't think that it was anything too serious at that time, but it very quickly grew into a complete inability to leave the home.

By the time she was nine years old, she was already spending 99.99 per cent of her time within the home and she appeared extremely depressed and withdrawn with very low self-esteem. By this stage we had withdrawn her from school, but the pressure that I had put on her to try to learn things and to be educated at home had only pushed her further away from me.

She had completely withdrawn from all social contact including that of her family. She was locked away in her own little world. Eventually she even found leaving home for fun activities and ones that she had personally chosen impossible. The more we offered, tried and tempted her, the more resistant and anxious she became. By the age of nine-and-a-half she was a complete recluse and she had also isolated herself from her family.

She would spend hour after hour, day after day absorbed in playing on her computer, iPad or watching TV. She was low, anxious, experiencing random but regular panic attacks, depressed, isolated, introverted and extremely volatile, angry and short-tempered. Her sleep became a real issue and was completely upside down. She would be awake all night and asleep all day.

Having a child with PDA is tough, challenging and mentally exhausting, but when you see your, previously challenging but happy child, reduced to a child who appears to be in the grips of a complete breakdown with none of the joy and laughter left in her soul, it is truly heart wrenching. My child with PDA had become crushed with trying to deal with and understand her condition, coupled with too many years of us trying to fix something that simply could not be fixed.

By understanding her and allowing her to be herself, while simultaneously building up her self-esteem and trying to gently undo the years of damage, our quirky little girl with an infectious laugh and a love for fun gradually began to return to us.

I initially tackled these issues by trying to repair my relationship with Mollie, because it had become very fraught and strained in the months leading up to and following removing her from school. I am the first to admit that my own exhaustion and depleting mental health would frequently mean that I was not in the best place to be a good parent for a child with PDA.

I really had to dig deep to make sure that I was adequately covering up and camouflaging any signs of my own ravaged mental health and the anxiety and depression that I also faced on a daily basis. It was time to deliver an Oscar-winning performance of happiness, contentment and joyfulness in the hope that she would pick up on and respond to the positive vibes that I was desperately trying to exude.

In conjunction with this, I dropped any attempts at learning and just allowed Mollie to follow her own agenda completely. There were no limits on screen time or obvious attempts from me to encourage her to come out of her solo world and interact.

Instead, following advice from a fellow parent, I would try to tempt her away from her isolated world by leaving appealing things to do around the house, for example baking packs in the kitchen, arts and crafts packs in her playroom, magazines in the lounge and so on. I would often sit near her and colour in or start making something, in the hope that she would join in. I was careful never to initiate or suggest interaction, because this would have immediately prompted avoidance. Instead I waited patiently and hoped that she would come to me.

Eventually, after a long, long time, she did start taking the bait and we gradually began to share pleasant times with each other. As our relationship improved and we spent more quality time together, she began opening up to me, now and again, about how she felt about herself and her life. I used these opportunities to reinforce how much we all loved her and that it was okay to be different. I explained that our lives may be different to what we see going on around us but that we needed to accept that difference and focus on what we could do rather than what we couldn't do.

Gradually, over a period of several months, Mollie began actively to seek out my company and she appeared to be far more accepting of herself; I hoped the self-loathing was beginning to disappear. This process of rediscovering each other and rebuilding our broken relationship went a long way to improving my own mental health as well. We were both travelling together to a far better place, both emotionally and mentally.

However, although she appeared to be improving emotionally, we still couldn't get Mollie to leave the home with any regularity, so we decided to focus on this aspect of her recovery.

As part of the healing process, Mollie had required a period of complete 'social detox', which we facilitated for her, during which time she could recuperate, regroup and rebuild. This is a radical approach and may only be needed for those who, like Mollie, appear to be on the extreme end of the spectrum. However I was becoming increasingly worried about her inability to go out and do anything at all. She appeared to be petrified of the outside world, and so I tentatively decided to try to tackle this issue.

Shortly before her tenth birthday I decided to try to broach the subject with her. It is very rare that she actually opens up or discusses anything, so what was to follow was a real breakthrough. I asked Mollie if she wanted to go out but couldn't or if she actually didn't want to go and just preferred to stay at home. It was important for me to make the distinction between the two; wanting to go out but being unable to do so is very different than simply not wanting to.

We then had one of those rare moments when she actually opened up to me. I can only tell the story from Mollie's point of view, and I am aware that the reasons behind her self-imposed exile may not be the same for other individuals with PDA. However, it may go some way to shedding some light on what may be behind the reclusive nature of some children with PDA.

MOLLIE'S REASONS FOR HER SELF-IMPOSED EXILE IN HER OWN WORDS

I can't go out because I am so scared of what may happen, what someone may say, even someone saying, 'Don't touch that,' scares me because I feel embarrassed that I have been told off. Then I feel like they will be watching me all day, waiting for me to do something else. I don't even like looking out of the window because I don't want anyone to see me. I just feel as if everyone's eyes are watching me all the time, waiting for me to do something wrong so that they can tell me off. I feel very frightened about doing things wrong or doing something stupid because being told off is so humiliating and embarrassing.

It is hard to leave the house because that in itself is a demand not to mention the huge anxiety that I feel because I don't know what will happen while I am out. It has been worse since I was held down at school when I was eight years old, it was terrible, and all I wanted to do was to be by myself to calm down.

My teachers wouldn't leave me alone, following me everywhere, watching me. I kicked out and ran away, I just wanted to sit on a bench by myself to calm down. When they caught me I was frightened and stressed because I just needed to be on my own but they held me down.

All my friends saw me being held down, the look on their faces, I can even remember now. The shame and the humiliation, how could I ever go back? Even when you arrived they wouldn't let me go so that I could run to you. I couldn't breathe; it was so scary and so awful. I often imagine that I'm in the school playground and the whole school witnesses me being held down.

I know that this won't happen when I go out with you but I always think about it. I can't explain why it stops me from going out; I know it doesn't make sense.

Mollie sobbed as she opened up about how deep rooted the results of her restraint had become and how it had affected her. The good news is that she said that she felt better for talking about it.

The school in question was and probably still is a wonderful school. The members of staff in question were fully supportive of Mollie and went to great lengths to understand and implement PDA strategies. I understand why they needed to restrain her; she was attacking a teacher and they were worried that she may run away from the school property leaving her vulnerable and in danger.

As soon as they had no option, other than to restrain her, the school called me and requested that I should go there immediately to support Mollie. If they had not responded as they did and she had run off and been knocked over by a car then I would have been the first person demanding to know how this could have been allowed to happen. So while I fully empathise with Mollie, I also understand the awful predicament that the school was in.

I suppose that what we can deduce from Mollie's insight and our knowledge of what drives her behaviour is that there are many factors at hand that may have worked together to lead her into complete isolation and depression.

- Leaving the home is in itself a demand.

- The uncertainty and unpredictability associated with human nature and what other people may say or demand always provokes huge anxiety.

- Not being intuitively aware of how you should behave, speak and interact with others in order to avoid slipping up and doing something that may prompt someone to correct you or tell you off.

- The exhaustion of trying to control this unpredictability by avoiding demands and being in control is exhausting, and experience may have taught her that this is not always a successful strategy.

- Being unable to navigate successfully the social highway while simultaneously dealing with high anxiety, embarrassment, failure and the loss of one friendship after another is bound to lead to low self-esteem and depression.

- Years of being completely misunderstood, feeling totally out of sync with the rest of the world and being forced, against her will, to behave in a way that simply wasn't possible for her all took their toll. The failure of her second school placement, being restrained and then being unable to cope at her third school placement really was the straw that broke the camel's back.

I think that it is also safe to say that the following quote from another parent of a child with PDA is very relevant and should be heeded: 'Socialising may be extremely important for the typically developing child but for a child with PDA the results of that social exposure can be TRAUMA!' (Parent of a child with PDA 2013).

It is so important to understand what drives any behaviour in order to help the individual concerned. In the case of Mollie refusing to go out, I needed to address the reasons behind that refusal and simply to accept that in the case of socialising, for my child with PDA, perhaps less is more.

Remaining in the safe bubble of home and periodically dipping her toes into the outside world may, for Mollie, be the optimum environment. While we wanted to ease the social anxiety that was consuming her, we decided that this may be best addressed by only encouraging Mollie to engage in tiny amounts of social exposure that she felt that she could manage.

We initially took really small baby steps and progress was painfully slow. We would be really happy if Mollie could simply manage to step outside the front door; a short walk would be an added bonus. I tried to encourage her to go to the cinema by reassuring her that she could come home at any time. Even if this resulted in us only making it as far as the car on the drive and then returning back to the safety of home, this was okay. This did bring us some very small results, but success really did ebb and flow and it was often a case of one step forward rapidly followed by two steps back.

Finally, at the age of ten Mollie was seen by a new psychologist at CAMHS to explore the possibility of ADHD. The result of the 'Connor's Questionnaire' (a diagnostic tool to assess for the likelihood of ADHD) indicated that Mollie did meet the threshold for possible ADHD and a new psychiatrist from our local health authority agreed to monitor any medication that Mollie may be prescribed by the out-of-area hospital.

Mollie was prescribed risperidone by a clinician at the out-of-area hospital. The immediate results were amazing: she wanted to go out to places, she could follow instructions and demands without flipping out and she appeared to have more control over her impulsive reactions to people.

However, she quickly began to suffer from a combination of severe side effects. She became very grey and her eyes were black underneath, she was exhausted all of the time and she began experiencing dizziness. In addition, she went off all of her food and couldn't face eating anything, claiming that everything tasted different. The most concerning side effect was that she became obsessed with and petrified of dying and she would spend hours crying, in complete panic and unable to be on her own at all. This took on the all too familiar form that I had so often seen in my husband – the obsessive thought of dying was very reminiscent of his OCD.

Due to these severe side effects and other complications, Mollie was taken off risperidone within a few weeks. What her short period on risperidone had done, however, was to open the door to the outside world and even when she came off it, the door to the outside world was left ajar.

With the failure of risperidone, Mollie was discharged from the out-of-area hospital and our local psychiatrist now took on her case. We began fluoxetine a few weeks later. This helped to reduce her constant high anxiety and she appeared to be able to go out a little more often with less of the accompanying anxiety.

With regard to the possibility of ADHD, Mollie's psychiatrist and psychologist felt that because some the features of PDA can be so similar to ADHD, it can make it extremely difficult to peel the two apart in order to accurately determine if Mollie has purely PDA or PDA and ADHD. They were both agreed to continue to monitor this with a view to considering ADHD medication in the future.

I am pleased to add that this psychologist and psychiatrist that I have currently been dealing with have been far more receptive, understanding and helpful than any who I have previously experienced within CAMHS. Perhaps some of this is down to my own calmer approach towards professionals now that the huge crisis and storm that we had been weathering has greatly subsided.

Although the demand avoidance associated with leaving the home still continues, it is to a much lesser degree. I am now satisfied that we have successfully addressed the other mental health issues that had been caused by her original issue of PDA. Mollie will never go out and socialise to the extent that other children do, but we do appear to have moved from complete isolation due to extremely high levels of social anxiety to PDA demand avoidance only.

The process of healing Mollie's self-esteem, improving emotional well-being and giving her the confidence to go out, if she chooses to do so, took a period of just over one year of complete unschooling, social detox and the additional help of medication.

The secret to dealing with all of the other issues that Mollie's central difficulty of PDA had caused was to provide a full and all-round package of support and help. We had to deal with the central issue of understanding and handling her PDA successfully while also delicately tackling the other mental health issues that PDA had caused.

Part 5

Learning to Interact in the Neurotypical World

15

Mollie Dips her Toes in the Outside World

By the age of ten-and-a half, following three years of using PDA strategies, just over a year of complete unschooling while simultaneously working on Mollie's PDA Plus and with the help of medication, we were beginning to make steady progress. Mollie was occasionally going to the pictures, bowling and parks. This seemed to give her the courage and the confidence to face 'the street'. Playing in the street with the other children who lived there had previously been an absolute disaster and had caused us our most problematic and stressful periods with Mollie. However, that was two years before, and it was interesting to see how she would cope now that she was older, had more awareness of her condition and had her anxiety a little bit more under control as a result of taking fluoxetine.

Everything started out well, and Mollie appeared to be coping with playing with other children and navigating the social highway of our little street. Unfortunately, within a very short time the all-too-familiar 'honeymoon period' came to an end and the usual cracks began to appear. She had been disrespectful and rude to two of my neighbours and she was experiencing numerous flair ups with her new friends.

These flair ups led to meltdowns, swearing in the street, crying and self-loathing. My own anxiety, and Lee's, began to rocket as we saw the pattern emerging. We were now constantly waiting for another knock at the door from an offended neighbour, the sound of Mollie's voice screaming obscenities in the street and the sound of the front door crashing open followed by a tear-stained child marching through the house throwing the nearest things to hand. In addition to dealing with Mollie's reactions to socialising, we had the added emotional stress of dealing with the embarrassment that goes hand in hand with having a child who is displaying anti-social and inappropriate behaviour in a public forum.

Also, our house seemed to have become the local youth club, and dealing with having our personal space constantly infiltrated by other children in a tense and emotionally charged atmosphere was not conducive to the sanctuary from the outside world that Lee and I needed our home to be.

It was time to make some plans, do some work and lay down some boundaries, because this situation was not going to improve without intervention. The question was, how on earth, were we going to do any of the above with a child who refused to follow any social guidelines or rules? It was certainly too much to tackle in one go, so we knew that we would have to take very small steps and try to tackle the different areas at a snail's pace in a very indirect, non-confrontational manner.

Mollie's new friends were three sisters from across the street, and they always came to play as a trio. As Mollie copes better on a one-to-one basis, this was a further complication for her from the off. Three children are far more stressful for her to deal with than one and the voices of three children also caused her to experience sensory overload due to her sensory issues around sound.

Mollie's large, well-equipped playroom was, of course, a magnet for other children. Consequently, all play dates – often lasting for the whole day on weekends and school holidays – were based at our house. Four girls running around the house, screaming, giggling, slamming doors, falling out and arguing is stressful enough, but is even more so when you are painfully aware of the volatile and impulsive nature of your own child and what she is capable of when she blows. In addition, the mess was indescribable and we were looking at somewhere in the region of two to three hours of tidying up just to get our house back in some sort of order following these play sessions. During holidays this was a daily occurrence.

House rules

We decided to start by trying to implement a few simple house rules to reduce the stress and anxiety that Lee and I had to deal with as a result of allowing our home to be an open house in order to assist Mollie socially.

Following a rather traumatic morning resulting in Mollie having a meltdown, things had reached a critical level. Not only were we becoming increasingly stressed by the infiltration of our home, but Mollie was becoming increasingly obsessed with the sisters. If they were going out somewhere then she would run into the house demanding to be taken to the same place as them at a millisecond's notice. As much as I love and want to accommodate my daughter's unique needs, there is only so much that Lee and I can do.

I have always had an open-house policy with my son and his friends. It was never really an issue and it was common for him to have four friends over for the day and for sleepovers. The difference, however, was that Jake and his friends never caused us a moment's stress and they all obeyed house rules and were always courteous.

With Mollie, it was a very different story – play dates were loud and stressful, Mollie showed no respect for us or our home. We also had to deal with the numerous rows, which could often spiral out of control with Mollie swearing, kicking off and saying hurtful things and, in the past, having violent outbursts towards her guests. The responsibility for the emotional well-being of other people's children was extremely stressful and on top of this, as a parent, I had to monitor how much exposure to certain behaviours was either fair or safe for the other children.

I informed Mollie that her dad and I were becoming increasingly stressed by the growing levels of high anxiety, problematic behaviour and impending meltdowns that her socialising was causing. My initial suggestion was that it might be better for all of us if she suspended socialising until she could deal with it a little bit better.

At this point she looked at me in sheer terror and exclaimed that she just couldn't bear the thought of being alone in the world again. My heart melted, so I asked Mollie if we could draw up a set of house rules that would be amenable to all of us and explained that she could have a major input in what these rules would be. She tearfully agreed that this would be a good idea, so our house rules were drawn up:

- The garage, which is carpeted and tidy, and the garden would be free for her and her friends to play in until midday. This would give me a few hours in the morning of having my home free and being able to get jobs done.

- Mollie's playroom would be open between the hours of midday and 5.00pm, but I did not want the girls running through the house so they were to stay in the playroom or her bedroom.

- At 5.00pm the playroom and bedroom access would close for the day, but the girls could still have access to the garage and the garden. This would allow me to tidy the playroom and her bedroom following their activities and give me a cut-off point when I knew that my home would belong to me again.

- At 7.00pm the Sherwin household would be closed and any further play would need to take place in the street.

We both negotiated and agreed to these arrangements and attached them to the fridge door with a magnet.

Mollie has courteously followed these guidelines since we made them, which, to some degree, lessened the stress on us because we all knew where we stood. Of course she will always push against and attempt to renegotiate these rules, and I try to be flexible during such periods, but it has given us a framework to work within.

Mollie also explained to me that she was worried that if she didn't give her friends full access to the house, follow them to places at their request or give them things (she had given one child her old bike) they wouldn't want to be friends with her. Her self-esteem and self-awareness regarding how difficult and complex she could be meant that she thought she could only attract friends if she had lots of things to offer other than herself. It was time to try to build up some of her depleted self-esteem. Mollie and I sat with a pen and paper and I asked her what all of her good qualities were. Between us we ascertained that Mollie is funny, bouncy, imaginative, quirky, good at making games up, good at arts and crafts and very loyal. We then wrote down a list of her not so positive attributes, which we all have, and we decided that Mollie could be bossy, controlling and stubborn and say mean things.

So she had seven positive points versus only four not-so-positive points. I informed Mollie that we all have less desirable aspects to our personalities, but as long as an individual's good points outweigh their negative points, they would always be a valued and sought-after friend on their own merit, without needing to buy friendships. This seemed to make sense to her and increased her self-confidence to a certain degree.

Unfortunately, during the course of the next couple of months Mollie began struggling more and more with the huge effort required to play with the sisters, which eventually resulted in her worst meltdown for over two years. She completely trashed the whole house. She only threw and upturned things that I could tidy away, so I kept my distance and allowed her to get on with it. My husband did not cope very well and he ignored all of the golden rules of how to handle a meltdown, so I ordered him out of the house until the situation had calmed down.

The meltdown was fast and furious but because I kept my distance and allowed her to go hell for leather, while also remaining vigilant that she wasn't endangering herself, it soon burnt out. When she stopped and slumped crying on the landing I approached her and asked if she wanted me to sit with her or go away.

She wanted me to sit with her and so I gave her a cuddle and told her that I understood why things had got too much. She whimpered that she just couldn't cope with the pressure of being made to play with three children, due to the sisters coming as a package and not being allowed any personal space to sort out any disagreements with any individual sister. 'It's just all too much I just couldn't cope with the situation anymore,' she cried. She apologised about all of the mess that she had made and said that she would help me to tidy up.

The following day the girls made up and Mollie went out to play. However, the meltdown incident was then compounded when one of my less understanding neighbours upset Mollie by talking to her, according to Mollie and her friend, in a very unkind way. This incident between the neighbour and Mollie appeared to be the final straw. Mollie withdrew back into her bubble and didn't go out for a week.

On a positive note, at least she was able to retreat before her inability to cope reached levels of magnitude proportions. The world is full of judgemental and less understanding people, so Mollie will have to learn to tolerate the fact that some people may not be very nice or accepting of her and to turn the other cheek and not care.

There is, of course, the additional possibility that going out may at times become a demand on her that she needs to have some control over by not always agreeing to go out to play. Other children knocking on your door and asking you to go out is, after all, a demand.

We began to notice that Mollie would frequently say to children who would knock for her that she wasn't coming out to play today only for her then to go out five or ten minutes later. The purpose of this was, of course, to avoid the initial demand made by the other child and to remain in control by going out to play in her own time and under her own steam.

Currently, Mollie appears to be self-monitoring quite well. Periods of playing out for several days are followed by periods of her retreating, chilling out and, I imagine, recovering. She does appear to be settling into a comfortable routine.

16

Strategies for Teaching the Social Laws and Customs Outside of the Family

Following Mollie and I jointly discussing, deciding on and implementing our house rules, it was time to think about how to cross the next hurdle. How could I sensitively broach the subject of Mollie reining in her natural behaviour when she was interacting with others outside of the home?

This was not going to be easy to approach, remedy or fix with a child who has an anxiety-driven need to avoid any rules or expectations that society or I stipulate. Simply asking her not to swear, to be respectful to adults and to behave in an age-appropriate manner are all demands that she would instinctively and compulsively need to avoid complying with. Head and brick wall are the terms that spring to mind!

So I thought and thought about how best to approach this situation and how to broach it with her. Eventually I decided to try to help her understand how neurotypical people (NTs for short) think and interact with each other. I was hopeful that if she could understand how and why

NTs interact and behave in the way that they do, she might then understand why her own behaviour could appear confusing and disrespectful to them.

I have to make adjustments to my own behaviour in order to interact successfully with Mollie and those adjustments are easier to make if you can understand why you have to make them. So I came up with a variety of strategies to try to help Mollie understand how her behaviour may be seen by others and why this may not be beneficial to her. I explained that the adjustments that she needed to make were not for the benefit of others or their feelings but were simply to make her life easier and her social interactions more successful. An impairment in empathy means that Mollie is not driven to change her behaviours simply for the purpose of others; she has to see something beneficial in it for herself and even then it can be a massive struggle for her to act accordingly.

Strategy one: Role play

I have found role play successful in trying to help Mollie see herself through another individual's eyes. This could be a successful vehicle to help Mollie to understand how she was making someone else feel or why other individuals were reacting negatively towards her.

We made role play fun and really sent up the people who we were playing, making caricatures out of them. I would often play the part of Mollie, sending her up something rotten, and she would play the part of the upset or offended person.

Being on the receiving end of her own behaviour did help Mollie to view it from another perspective. This, of course, would not cure the issue of needing to avoid the correct behaviour that society dictates but it did at least teach her how other people are affected by her own behaviour, even though by her own admission, she didn't care.

I attempted to help her to realise that pretending to care and adjusting some aspects of her behaviour would have nothing but positive effects for her. Being good and charming can, after all, bring about even more control than simply refusing to conform.

Strategy two: Understanding why the Neurotypical brain and the PDA brain clash and developing tolerance for a different way of thinking from both sides

In order to assist Mollie to navigate the Neurotypical (NT) world as successfully as possible, we decided to try to fathom out the mysteries of NT social interaction. Just what does go on in the NT mind and why does it appear to react so adversely to the PDA mind? I would like to point out that neither mind is superior; they are different but equal.

Our home is Mollie's PDA world; this is where she can fully and truly be herself without the need to moderate, apologise or adapt her behaviour. People entering our PDA world are expected to accept, respect and try to understand Mollie for who she is and not to expect her to be any different.

Therefore, it stands to reason that if Mollie wants to dabble in the NT world, she will need to show the NTs the same respect. She will need to accept, respect and to try to understand the NTs. I don't see this as changing who you are so that you can fit in; I simply see it as respecting somebody else's laws, customs and traditions.

If she can learn to moderate her less desirable behaviours, which may be made easier by understanding how the NT mind functions, then she can, I hope, enjoy friendships and say goodbye to isolation. I will, of course, be simultaneously trying to also educate any new NTs who she is in contact with about how her mind works. I hope that somewhere in the middle we may be able to find a happy medium.

Clash of two different minds: point one

NTs rarely actually say exactly what is on their mind, which can be confusing for Mollie because her brain appears to do this naturally. NTs are constantly worrying and thinking about what they say and how they say it so that they don't upset, bore or annoy the other person. Because this comes natural to NTs it can be very confusing and shocking for them when Mollie doesn't show the same respect for their feelings and just blurts stuff out. NTs may wrongly assume that she is not a very nice person, which may be very hurtful for Mollie, especially when she may not understand why they think this about her or intuitively know what she has said wrong.

Advice for both mindsets

NTs – please try to be tolerant and to not take offence at Mollie's forthright way of saying things just like it is. Mollie may not intentionally be trying to shock, hurt or upset you; it is sometimes simply a case of her not truly understanding how these words may feel for you. Mollie may simply not be blessed with the same amount of natural intuitive instinct and empathy that you are. This doesn't mean that she is uncaring; it just means that her awareness of somebody else's feelings in relation to her own actions may not be as finely tuned as yours.

On the other side of the fence, words can really hurt so I encourage Mollie to think about how much words can often hurt her. I explain that although it is okay to be herself and to say what is on her mind, it also doesn't hurt to try to 'not say' hurtful things to people if she is aware of how those words can hurt. I explain that if she isn't sure if the words may hurt another person to imagine how she would feel if those words were said to her!

Clash of two different minds: point two

NTs naturally know and understand their pecking order in society and will automatically be inclined to show adults and authority figures respect. Mollie does not appear to have this natural instinct and finds it difficult to understand why she should be treated and expected to behave differently than adults.

From her point of view if it's okay for adults to swear, be in control, give orders and do what they want when they want, then why should it be different for her? Mollie may therefore expect to be shown the same respect and to be allowed to have the same freedom as adults and may talk to adults as equals.

This can be very confusing for NTs because in their culture children should be compliant, accept rules without question, not answer adults back and basically just do as they are told. Therefore, Mollie may simply be viewed by the NT as defiant, rude and out of control. Also, Mollie may, due to not knowing intuitively how to behave in relation to others, mirror the behaviour of adults thinking that this must be the correct way to behave because that is what she witnesses going on around her.

A child behaving like an adult and applying rules to other children when she ignores those very rules herself can appear extremely confusing. However isn't this exactly what we, as adults, often do on a daily basis? Adults teach children not to swear and react with horror when they do, but then, in complete contradiction, will often swear themselves. We tell children off for arguing with each other, making a mess, being short-tempered or having an off day, but aren't we all guilty of these crimes? In short, adults may often place much higher levels of expectation on children than they expect from fellow adults or from themselves. This is very confusing to Mollie – 'Do as I say and not as I do' is a term that will make little sense to Mollie and understandably so! She probably mimics the behaviour that she observes in adults and so she may not understand why this is then deemed inappropriate.

Advice for both mindsets
NTs – please try to understand that Mollie may not mean to be rude or disrespectful, it is just that in her world this pecking order doesn't exist. When your mind is wired for everyone to be equal and treated the same regardless of age, it is really confusing to be expected to be subservient simply because you are young. NTs' brains are wired to accept their pecking order in society without any undue stress or embarrassment. For Mollie, this aspect of the wiring process is very different and being expected to behave and to be treated so unequally can feel deeply unfair, stressful, embarrassing and humiliating.

On the other side of the coin, I suggest to Mollie that perhaps she can try to meet the NTs halfway so that it isn't such a shock to their delicate systems. I also suggest that if she is playing out, perhaps she can mirror some of the behaviour of other children and how they interact with adults. I emphasise that I don't mean for her to stop being who she naturally is, but simply to try to talk respectfully to other people without shouting or being rude.

I explain that falling out with a peer and telling them to 'shut up' or getting extremely annoyed with them is an occurrence that naturally happens between children and adults alike. However, if you, as a child, conduct yourself like that with an NT adult it may be too much for them to accept. I further explain that by toning the natural her down just a little bit, it may help her to keep these adults on side and this would ultimately be beneficial for her. If NT adults like you, they will want their kids to play with you. Being nice, even when you don't think you should be, can be a good way to keep things within your control!

Clash of two different minds: point three

'I needed to have a big reaction so that he could really see how upset I was. If I don't show it in an over-the-top way then he will never understand', explained Mollie following an incident with a neighbour when she had behaved disrespectfully.

This statement suddenly made a lot of sense to me, especially as it was a feature that I had previously noticed in Mollie. I only ever seem to get a response of sorrow or guilt from her when I either breakdown or explode. A big reaction from me is the only time that I see a positive reaction of recognition of my feelings in Mollie's response.

Mollie's statement and my observations indicated to me that in order for Mollie to really understand if someone was dissatisfied with her, she would need a big reaction from another person. Therefore, she has accepted this as a standard form of communication and feels that if she needs to adequately make her point, it needs to be done in an over-the-top and dramatic fashion.

She doesn't appear to register subtle or normal reactions, so she may assume that other people are the same. She needs points to be made in a loud and obvious fashion, so this is how she delivers her points to other people, under the assumption that they need the same approach.

Of course, this can cause a huge amount of misunderstanding. NTs may feel that their feelings and needs are often ignored by Mollie, and she may be confused as to why her loud and direct approach is met with such negative responses. This is a serious case of crossed wires.

Advice for both mindsets

NTs – Mollie may not necessarily pick up on the subtle clues that you pick up on, which is why she may only appear to react to strong reactions. But strong, loud or angry verbal reactions are likely to evoke high anxiety and stress in Mollie and are also likely to prompt an aggressive response. So it may be wise to explain how you feel with explanatory language while also keeping calm, for example, 'Those words hurt me so much that I am crying inside and my heart is breaking, even though you can't see it on the outside that is how I am feeling on the inside.' Keeping a calm voice but explaining with descriptive terms that Mollie can relate to may help her to understand how stressed or upset her behaviour is making you.

I discuss with Mollie how NTs can instinctively pick up if she is upset, angry, happy or nervous and that they will try to help and to adjust their behaviour according to how she is feeling. I tell her that if they don't pick up on how she is feeling, she can simply tell them and they will understand and try to help. NTs don't need to see big and dramatic reactions in order to be able to understand a situation. In fact, big and dramatic reactions can frighten NTs or make them feel angry.

Strategy three: Teaching social skills

I also decided to research how to teach empathy for children with ASD in the hope that I may be able to teach Mollie how to learn empathy and how to react appropriately at an intellectual level. I came across a wonderful website – Autism Teaching Strategies, that has lots of free downloads, videos and activities, and can be found in the list of useful resources in Appendix 3.

I couldn't have even attempted doing anything like this a year or even six months ago but I was hopeful that this may be the right time. I watched all of the videos by myself, made files on my computer and meticulously downloaded any activities that I thought could be helpful.

The more I can learn, know and have printed off, ready to use at a moment's notice, the more chance I have of slipping bits of learning in here and there. As we now all know, a direct approach will not be successful; I will have to keep on my toes and think of a variety of ways to introduce very small amounts of these activities at the very few and rare opportunities that she is open and receptive to listening.

I enjoyed a quick moment of success in enticing her to watching a few of the videos and taking part in some of the activities. The videos are mainly cognitive behaviour therapy videos about replacing negative thoughts with positive ones. They are very much based around ASD thoughts that I recognise so much in both of my children.

I purposefully watched these within earshot of Mollie while simultaneously laminating and cutting out the accompanying thought bubbles to the videos. I told Mollie that I was giving Jake some 'ASD lessons' to help him when he leaves school next year. She became jealous saying that I must love Jake more than her. I told her that she was more than welcome to have some ASD lessons too and that she could share Jake's downloaded and laminated activities.

She then sat down and watched the first four videos and helped me to cut out the thought bubbles. She really resonated with the thought and feeling videos and we laughed at how they related to her and Jake. So by hook or by crook, lesson one was achieved. When the next one occurs is anybody's guess but at least I am prepared with an armoury of strategies.

It's all a learning curve and it's all unchartered territory. We shall continue and see where our journey takes us. Today's small successes could well be tomorrow's failures, but at least we have tried and we have enjoyed a degree of success even if it only lasts for one day.

Strategy four: Appealing

I also appeal to Mollie to try to keep her behaviour in check when she is playing out. I must stress that I appeal rather than directly tell her. I always try to emphasise the positives that she will experience if she can manage to do it. If she can't, there will be natural consequences and it is these natural consequences that I hope will allow her to achieve, when possible, a degree of control over her social interactions and behaviours.

The more she manages to cope responsibly in the outside world, the more benefits she will reap. By the same token, if she continues to behave exactly as she wants, she will experience negatives. I have no control over who other parents will or won't allow their children to play with, so Mollie will need to be able to moderate some of her less desirable behaviours if she wants her current progress within this area to continue.

I feel that I have done my best and I really don't know what more that I can do at this time in order to encourage her to behave in ways that won't be offensive to others. Ultimately, the rest will be up to her, and she may need to take a few more hard knocks before she fully learns that certain behaviours need to be toned down.

Following this period of social education Mollie did not have any more run-ins with neighbours that were a result of her behaving inappropriately. However, we sadly did have a couple of neighbours who didn't appear to understand how they should behave in relation to her. This was despite my many conversations with them, and it would cause Mollie difficulties even when she was trying her best and not behaving inappropriately towards them. Unfortunately this is 'life' and I have learned that there is no use knocking if there is no one in, so we shall just have to cross those bridges as and when we reach them.

Part 6

Entering the Adolescent Years and Looking to Adulthood

17

Periods and Puberty

So Far, So Good

Although this is an area that we have only recently begun to experience, hence the incredibly short chapter, I am pleased to report: so far, so good. Although Mollie is still only ten years old, puberty has begun and we really haven't noticed any difference in Mollie as a result. She has taken it in her stride and has not been at all concerned about the changes that her body is going through. Of course this will be different for every child but for us it does all seem to be going fairly smoothly.

I was rather caught out and surprised when she recently began her periods. This was totally unexpected, because I did not feel that her body had gone through enough changes to warrant me beginning to worry about her starting her periods. Consequently, I had not had the chat with her and it came as a shock for all concerned.

I didn't want to discuss this too early with her in case the thought of it freaked her out and caused her months of unnecessary worrying. I had decided to wait until nearer the time so that I could eliminate a period of stress, waiting and a big build-up, as this can often increase anxiety and behaviours. Unfortunately, my timing was off and we were both caught off guard.

However when the fateful day did arrive she simply took it in her stride. Following the initial horror of wondering what on earth was going on, she was absolutely cool. She already understands and knows about sex, thanks to a full and frank initiation from boys at her third school placement, and how babies are made, so it was relatively straightforward to explain to her what a period was and why it was happening.

I provided her with some sanitary towels and showed her how to use them, which she was absolutely fine with. Because Mollie experiences demand avoidance over flushing the loo, I had been particularly dreading this time and had wondered how she would cope with the hygiene aspect. However, if she was out playing she would come in to check if she needed to change. She did ask how long she was going to have to put up with this for, and so she wasn't too pleased when I told her about a week every month for the next 40 years or so.

My sister asked me if I had noticed whether Mollie had experienced pre-menstrual tension (PMT). 'How the hell would I know?' I replied – as far as I'm concerned she's been premenstrual for the last ten years, how would I notice any difference? In true Mollie style, she wasn't the least bit embarrassed by recent events and proceeded to tell anyone and everyone that she had started her periods. She appeared to be very proud of herself and enjoyed bragging about it.

18

Children with PDA Grow into Adults with PDA

I think that it is so important to highlight that PDA is not a condition that only affects children. The fact that it is only recently being more recognised and diagnosed means that there must be a massive community of undiagnosed adults, as well as the small numbers of adults with PDA who were diagnosed when they were children.

Virtually all of the current research, support (such as it is), strategies, awareness and diagnostic developments seem to be geared towards children only. But what about the children of yesteryear who are now adults, don't they deserve the same recognition and support as our children do? After all, today's children will be tomorrow's adults and unless we tackle both areas for increased awareness, our children may be left high and dry when the time comes for them to move from children's services to adult services.

The term PDA was first coined in the 1980s, so those early children that were first identified are now adults with PDA. Follow-up studies on those individuals showed that the PDA profile endured over time and continued into adulthood and was, therefore, a lifelong condition

(Newson and David, 1999). The findings of this study were discussed by Christie *et al.*:

> Individuals with PDA and their families will need support throughout their lives. Parents' fears for the future mirror those of parents of children with other ASDs, but may be magnified by the variable recognition and understanding of the condition and some of the particular challenges in behaviour that persist for some young people with PDA. Parents express worries about their children's needs, about 'falling through the net' of those services provided for people with learning disabilities and mental health, about them getting into trouble with the criminal justice system, about not having enough support to live independently, about the demands placed on them and other family members as carers, and about what will happen to their son or daughter when they are no longer able to provide them with support. (Christie *et al.* 2011, p.193)

Because PDA is a spectrum condition with individuals affected to varying degrees, I suppose that the long-term prognosis for individuals will vary depending on how severely their PDA affects them and on how much suitable support they receive both growing up and into adulthood, as discussed by Christie *et al.*:

> PDA, like other conditions within the autism spectrum, is a life-long condition that can have enormous impact on the opportunities of the person affected and cause massive problems for the family, both practically and emotionally. At the same time a better understanding of the distinctive profile and needs of children with PDA is gradually emerging and, with it, a greater recognition of which provision and approaches and are most needed and effective. (Christie *et al.* 2011, p.194)

Some self-diagnosed adults, and some of those who were diagnosed as children, are gradually finding their way to the online support groups. Through these support groups it would appear that some adults with a PDA diagnosis from childhood are ignored by local services and do not receive any help or support during adulthood. Adults without a diagnosis have nowhere to turn to for an assessment, as there are currently no officially recognised organisations offering an assessment and diagnostic service for adults.

From my experience of the support groups and from discussions with adults with diagnosed or suspected PDA, some adults with PDA may be able to work to varying degrees – a few may be able to hold down a job but others may have a history of having numerous jobs, unable to stick at any one job for very long. There are also a considerable amount of individuals for whom work just isn't a viable option or a realistic possibility.

The parents of these individuals may still be responsible for many aspects of their son's or daughter's day-to-day living, for example cleaning, cooking, ironing, tidying and so on. Some individuals with PDA have tried to live independently but have had to return home because they have not been able to cope mentally with all of the demands associated with independent living.

Many parents may be entering old age still providing high levels of support for their adult children without any help from the authorities. Some adults with PDA may have managed to maintain a relationship and possibly even have had children but may struggle with day-to-day living without the support of their partner. These relationships may place a great deal of strain on the partner, who may find himself or herself in the role of a carer. Due to the lack of recognition and understanding of adults with PDA, there is a complete lack of support, and in many cases no support at all, for individuals with PDA, their families, partners and carers.

In order to improve the current situation for adults with PDA first and foremost, the adult PDA community desperately needs a recognised assessment and diagnostic service. It is also vitally important that support services acknowledge the huge need for individuals with PDA to be able to access the correct services throughout their life, because this is a lifelong condition.

Supporting adults with PDA could take various forms. Adults could be assisted to live independent lives by being offered support for things that many adults with PDA struggle with, like cleaning and cooking meals. An outreach service would be invaluable for an adult with PDA and would provide the individual with the reassurance of knowing that they have someone to call upon to assist with any on-going issues or for some much-needed company. An outreach service may also reduce the pressure on carers and give them another person to lean on or to ask advice from. Even simple services like offering assistance in filling out forms would be extremely valuable and useful for many adults with PDA. I also feel that adults with PDA would find professional help from experienced clinical practitioners, such as psychologists and psychiatrists, extremely useful. Following a diagnosis, it is essential that these individuals are helped to understand themselves and receive aftercare and support so that they are better able to navigate the social highway.

I can't help but wonder if the adults who are finding their way to the PDA community are the ones who have, for whatever reason, fared the best with a very complex condition. I do worry about how life may have turned out for some of the other children, and their families, who grew into adulthood without ever having received either a diagnosis or support. Knowing how challenging it can be to raise a child with PDA, I worry about how many children may have eventually, as a last resort, been placed in care by distraught parents simply unable to cope anymore.

Being raised in care is not the most desirable environment for any child, so I can't even begin to contemplate how this environment may affect the long-term prognosis for an individual with undiagnosed PDA. I also wonder how families cope, in the long term, without an understanding of why their child behaves the way that they do and without knowing the correct strategies. The answer to this is, of course, unknown and we can only speculate:

- Without the correct strategies from parents, do some of these undiagnosed children continue to have violent meltdowns and rages, often aimed at their parent, as they grow into adulthood?

- Do some of these children grow up to be deeply disturbed adults who are often in trouble with the police and are in and out of prison on a regular basis?

- How many of these undiagnosed adults suffer from crippling mental health issues leading to self-harm and substance abuse?

- Or is the worst-case scenario the possibility that undiagnosed children with PDA may grow into adults who exhibit all of the above?

There is currently only one published paper that delves into this area (Eaton and Banting 2012), and it does offer some insight into the possible eventual outcome of some individuals with undiagnosed PDA. The paper identifies that many patients in residential and secure settings have no formal diagnosis of autism but may in fact be on the spectrum. It also seeks to outline the diagnosis and subsequent treatment and intervention planning for a young woman in a low secure hospital. It summarises the literature in relation to the diagnosis of PDA in children and describes how this diagnosis may present in adults. Due to the lack of literature available about either the clinical presentation or management guidance of PDA (an atypical presentation of autism spectrum disorder) in adults, a case study on this young woman is used in the paper. The paper concludes that the lack of an appropriate diagnosis and inappropriate formulation of the underlying causes of challenging behaviour can lead to patients becoming impossible to manage and that many may benefit from diagnosis and autism-specific intervention. It also highlights the challenges of adult diagnosis of autism in highly complex individuals and outlines novel approaches to treatment.

It is important to raise awareness and recognition of PDA in both children and adults. Improved understanding, management and support can lead to better outcomes for the attainments, prospects and emotional well-being for all those affected by the condition.

Part 7

How PDA has Affected Our Family

19

Family Dynamics

The dynamics of every family are different and this will affect how the family as a whole copes and deals with 'living with PDA'. There isn't a right or a wrong way; it is simply a case of finding the best way for you and your family.

I can only speak from my own personal experiences and how our family has coped and adjusted to the needs of two complex children one of whom has PDA.

Work and careers

The arrival of a child with PDA can cause drastic changes in finance. Often it can be impossible for both parents to continue working due the amount of time that may be spent either at meetings, appointments or home with a child who has either been suspended, excluded or is school refusing.

In addition, mental health issues that can affect carers may mean that they become unable to work, regardless of any improvements at home, due to nerves, stress, depression and high anxiety. Living with PDA has changed who I am and my personality to the very core. I gave up work because I really had no choice due to Mollie's continual school refusal.

I didn't just go to work as a means of earning money; I actually loved my job. I started work in the family business (a carpet and bed retail outlet) when I was 18 years old as the tea girl, cleaner and office administrator. As the years went by, I educated myself on every aspect of the business. I had discovered my niche – I thrived on the challenge of buying in the right stock, calculating profit margins, advertising and even teaching myself how to do my own VAT returns, calculating my profit on return and working out the business's breakeven figures.

My dad eventually retired and I was left to oversee the general running of the carpet shop; the day-to-day running was left to two very loyal, honest and exceptionally good members of staff. My sister (who had just joined the business) and I co-owned and ran our new venture, a large specialist retail bed outlet. My dad had negotiated the rent and designed the structural layout and I did the rest to set the business up, buying in the stock, layout, pricing, advertising, business stationery and so the list goes on.

By this time I had invested over 20 years of my life in the family business and I had gone from being the tea girl to running the whole lot. What I am trying to emphasise here is that giving up my career was not a decision that I would have chosen to make because I just didn't want to go to work anymore. I had no choice; giving up my career was a sacrifice and not one that I actually wanted to make.

The minute Mollie started a new school placement, people would ask me, 'Are you going back to work now?' Well, the answer to that was that, although I loved my job and thrived in the environment and the challenges that it created, I didn't think that I could ever cope with the demands of work again. My nerves are always on edge, my confidence is very low, but steadily improving, and my ability to handle pressure, cope with the general public, instinctively deal with on-the-spot problems and multitask in a public forum like the workplace are things that I just don't think I would be able to cope with mentally or handle effectively anymore.

I am very lucky that the family business can still support me, but I also hate this because I have always been fiercely independent and proud to be so. I don't receive any benefits other than Disability Living Allowance (DLA) or state handouts, but I do have to rely on family handouts. Contrary to how carers of challenging children may often be portrayed by certain quarters of the general public, being unable to work and reliant on others is not desirable or pleasant.

I am exceptionally lucky that our finances have not been drastically affected. I can't imagine coping with the stress of being in financial difficulties on top of everything else. Unfortunately, many families are not as lucky as ours and may potentially suffer extreme financial difficulties as a result of supporting their child with PDA. However, this is not always the case and many parents of children with PDA do continue to support themselves, although this will be dependent on the severity of the PDA, the mental health of the parents and the dynamics of the family.

My ASD family
Our family consists of one dad aged 46 (ASD/Asperger's, OCD), one mum aged 43 (stressed but no other formal diagnosis), one son aged 15 (ASD/Asperger's) and one daughter aged 10 (ASD/PDA). Ours is probably quite a familiar family unit within the ASD world. When a child is identified as having an ASD – in our case this was

Mollie – the parents may realise when they are studying the subject that this condition also accurately describes either themselves or other family members and explains the difficulties and/or mental health issues that may have plagued those individuals for a lifetime. You already know about Mollie, but here is a little bit of information about Jake and Lee.

Jake

Mollie's original diagnosis was Asperger's and so I read and watched everything that I could get my hands on about Asperger's. The more I read, the less I saw an accurate description that reflected Mollie. However, the profile and the associated difficulties went a long way to accurately describing my son. I had always known that his behaviours and his way of seeing the world appeared odd, and he had at various times also suffered from huge tantrums, meltdowns, terrible anxiety, phobias, obsessions, motor and vocal tics, taking things literally, misinterpreting sarcasm, routines and struggling to maintain friendships.

I had taken him to the doctors and to CAMHS on numerous occasions from the age of two but I had never got anywhere with regard to his underlying difficulties other than, 'Yep you've guessed it', our parenting and the offer of parenting courses. From the minute he was born he never stopped screaming and his challenging behaviour was, during certain stages in his early years, worse than Mollie's!

From when he was about eight I really began to parent him differently. Looking back, I was using ASD strategies without knowing it. From this age, a lot of his explosive behaviour disappeared and was replaced with more internalised behaviour in the form of anxiety and emotional problems.

My son required extremely careful handling and I invested huge amounts of time in trying to understand and reach him, research techniques that may help him and so on. One of the hardest things was simply building a relationship with him, because a typical relationship between Jake and his family members just didn't come naturally. It had to be created, invested in, maintained and allowed to grow over time.

Discovering Asperger's when Jake was 11 and finally understanding how he saw the world was the final piece of the jigsaw puzzle for us and our son. I decided to pursue a formal assessment for him and he was assessed by our ASD diagnostic team following a battle with CAMHS.

His assessment for Asperger's concluded that he did not have Asperger's, but instead had ASD traits and severe anxiety. When I questioned this and explained all of the current issues that I was going through and that I didn't agree with their findings, I was informed that perhaps Jake was saying that he was too stressed to attend school because he was copying Mollie and that they really didn't understand why a diagnosis was so important to me! It was during this discussion that I realised how little these professionals appeared to know about ASD as a whole rather than just at a surface level.

When Jake started senior school, his anxiety and inability to cope absolutely peaked. Both he and his dad had found the recent house move almost unbearable due to the change and had both suffered months of extreme anxiety in anticipation, not knowing how they would cope with such a drastic change. It was just too much for Jake to deal with. Eventually he was too ill to attend school and had a month at home while I tried to think about how to solve the situation. Jake's school was, at that time, very supportive and we eventually agreed that it would be beneficial for Jake to attend on a part-time basis until he was ready to resume a full-time timetable.

Fast forward a few years and Jake was, again, experiencing difficulties, bouts of depression and anxiety. I had resisted revisiting Asperger's, because any battle left in me had become increasingly thin on the ground. However I eventually decided to pursue this again, because a diagnosis, I had long since realised, was the only way to receive the necessary support, understanding and tolerance of others.

Jake was, at the age of 14, eventually diagnosed with Asperger's by an experienced and well-respected clinician. At last I had closure and the correct diagnosis, support and understanding for all of my family. Unfortunately I had been required to pay privately for each one, amounting to a cost of approximately £3750!

We have made really good progress with Jake and he is now doing extremely well. He is very high functioning and with the correct support and guidance he has learnt so much, at an intellectual level, that his Asperger's can go by unnoticed to many people.

Lee

During the period that I was studying Asperger's, I also began to see lots of traits in my husband who had been plagued with mental health issues from the age of 16. He couldn't really remember his early childhood, so I spoke to his auntie and the description that she gave me of my husband as a boy was a carbon copy of my son. In addition to his similarities to Jake, he had also been a regular school runner and he was seen by a child physiologist in the 1970s when he was 11 years old.

He had spent his teenage years rebelling against authority, being disruptive in school, fighting, smoking cannabis and dabbling in petty crime until he eventually got into trouble with the police. This was a defining moment for him and was when he made the decision to really try and turn his life around.

Taking up martial arts was instrumental because he respected his teachers and he had to be disciplined, fit and focused. This sport also enabled him to release all of his adrenaline and anger in a safe and controlled environment. One of Lee's greatest traits is that when he sets his mind to something he throws himself into it to an obsessive level. His ethos is that it isn't good enough to be good, he has to be the best and nothing short of that will do. Martial arts was a lifesaver and gave him exactly what he needed just at the right time, stopping his slide down a very slippery slope.

Lee is now, and has been since the age of about 20, a very straight-laced, law-abiding citizen. He successfully runs his own business. However he is plagued, even to this day, with mental health issues, namely his OCD.

Lee was diagnosed with OCD at the age of 33 and at the age of 43 he was also diagnosed with Asperger's following a private referral. This diagnosis answered so many questions for both of us and saved our marriage.

Prior to his diagnosis, my husband was obsessed with himself, his interests and his life. My life and needs never seemed to crop up in his head and I was more like his mother than his wife. I cared for him, cleaned for him, looked after him and nursed him through his mental health issues without ever receiving any emotional or practical support in return. He never sought out my company or wanted to spend time with me; he just wanted to either live on his computer or be out pursuing his interests and hobbies. I felt very lonely and taken for granted in this marriage.

Lee was happy with our relationship, so he couldn't understand why I wasn't. He was out every night and most Saturdays pursuing his own interests while I was working full time and single handedly rearing two very difficult and challenging children. However, once Jake was old enough to enjoy football and speedway this did only leave me with Mollie on a Saturday.

His mind had just never intuitively viewed life from my side of the fence and I had always assumed that he was a very selfish, self-centred individual who sulked like a child if he was expected to do anything that didn't revolve around him. It was only about four years ago, following our discovery and understanding of Asperger's, that my rather useless and self-absorbed husband transformed into Wonder Dad and Super Hubby; better late than never I suppose, and he was worth waiting for.

Because of his diagnosis I can better understand his needs and why he can't cope with certain things like 'change' or not being able to obsessively follow an interest or hobbies and why he may often appear to show no care or thought for me. It isn't that he is uncaring or thoughtless, just that he doesn't always intuitively think about how his actions may impact on others. He has been able to learn to put himself in my shoes at an intellectual level, so that he can understand why I need support or why I may get upset at certain things.

The last three years has seen our marriage go from the verge of collapse to a strong, supportive unit. Having a child with PDA can cause many marriages to split up and I can understand why. The stress of trying to cope can make you lash out at each other and you can often have different ideas on how the behaviour should be dealt with.

Fortunately, for us, Mollie's difficulties led us to ASD, which in turn helped our son, my husband and ultimately our whole family to all understand and tolerate each other in a way that we never could before. Mollie having PDA and the huge challenges that it brings also pushed my husband and I together.

We are the only ones who can truly understand what the other one is going through and support each other through it. Other than my parents, no one else could ever be able to empathise or understand the extremes that our lives took.

This really forged a strong unit based on support, love, respect and friendship. Lee is now a partner who stands shoulder to shoulder with me and shares the physical and emotional workload. He still enjoys his football and coaching my son's football team, but he has reined in all of his solo pursuits so that he can actively and fully support his family.

Siblings

Jake and Mollie don't really have much of a brother–sister relationship but as well as the obvious difficulties they have, they are different genders with different interests and there is a five-year age gap. This is probably completely normal for most siblings of their age and perhaps this will change as they get older because they do love each other, they just don't understand each other.

Jake quite reasonably finds it very difficult to understand and to cope with Mollie's complex and challenging personality. Because his views can be very black and white and rigid, it is not easy for him to be able to comprehend fully the driving force behind Mollie's difficulties.

Mollie gets very frustrated with Jake because she can't understand why he isn't like the big brothers that she sees on American sitcoms with extremely animated, exaggerated facial expressions and a larger-than-life personality. She wants him to smile more, laugh more, stop looking so serious and give her hugs and loves. Unfortunately Mollie's 'ideal' of a good brother and his presentation of Asperger's don't quite go together and she has huge difficulty in understanding why Jake does not 'naturally' do these things.

Coping with two children with different variations of ASD growing up was challenging to say the least. However it did bring us some advantages and was only a problem during the years that both children needed parental supervision. For these seven years – fortunately it wasn't longer – if I was meeting the needs of one child, it would ultimately be infringing on the needs of the other. By the time Jake was 12, these types of issues began to fade away. However, until then it was extremely hard work and stressful. I never seemed to have two happy children at the same time. If one was happy, the other one would invariably be kicking off. An example of this was when Jake went through a phase of really struggling to go out anywhere and wanted to be on his Xbox 24/7. This was due to a combination of anxiety in social situations and wanting to pursue his current obsession. It could be extremely difficult to negotiate with him or for him simply to accept going to the park for an hour after school. Everything was very black and white and it was very difficult to get him to see anything from anybody else's perspective. Following a school pickup, which held its own unique PDA challenges, meltdowns, kick-offs and Mollie randomly attacking other children to name but a few, I would eventually make it to the park, usually stressed and frazzled by this stage, only to then have a standoff with my son.

Often he would point-blank refuse to go to the park and would simply sit down wherever we were and refuse to move. Other times he may endure the visit, sitting next to me permanently, refusing to engage with the social advances that his classmates made towards him while retaining a very solemn expression and periodically hitting himself on the side of the head. Every two minutes he would mumble. 'I want to go home now.' Meanwhile, Mollie would probably be reaching meltdown status as she desperately tried to completely control and dominate every child in the park! I would also be on edge wondering which child she would lash out at first.

On paper this may just sound like the normal, run-of-the-mill difficulties of coping with two children, however it is important to understand the intensity, frequency and duration of these encounters. This type of difficulty was a constant thread through our lives because Jake did not want to go anywhere and, at that stage, Mollie wanted to be out all day every day. It is ironic that only a few years later the reverse would be true. Fortunately, Jake had then reached an age where he could go out by himself with friends and so we could happily accommodate Mollie's needs.

Jake does not have PDA but as a younger child he could be highly avoidant of doing anything that either caused him anxiety or that he did not see as being personally advantageous for him. His avoidance was not as extreme as Mollie's and he behaved in different ways but it was far more than you would expect to see in a NT child. During these daily episodes he could not be motivated by the use of rewards or punishments to engage in social experiences.

He found them too stressful and uncomfortable and he derived no personal fulfilment from them.

If I had only had one child, during this stage, life would have been so much easier for all of us. It would have enabled me to completely and utterly meet the individual needs of my child regardless of whether they wanted to stay in or go out. As it was I had two children who both had great difficulty in complying with anything that they didn't want to do; obviously in Mollie's case this was far more extreme. In addition to this, they were both inflexible, rigid and had difficulty adjusting their own needs in order to accommodate the needs of anyone else.

Because I had two children and there was only one of me, each child had invariably to accommodate the needs of the other. By the time one of them had backed down, we would have experienced numerous meltdowns and explosions. Life was much easier at weekends when Lee was at home. Once Jake was old enough, he spent Saturdays at football and speedway with his dad. On Sundays, Lee and I would split and have one child each. It was the school run and the school holidays that were the hardest to cope with.

In order to try to minimise this issue I would, when possible, ask my parents to have Jake when Mollie wanted to go out and school pickups quickly became a two-man job. These types of issues naturally faded out as Jake grew older and could be left without parental supervision. There were also lots of other difficulties, but this was perhaps one of the main ones for us.

I definitely see a big advantage, from my point of view, that my child with PDA was my younger child. Although Jake had his own difficulties and issues, a five-year age gap did help with the difficulties associated with Mollie. As he has grown older, he has been able to understand and accommodate her far more than a younger child would have been able to, but perhaps he can't be as flexible as an older NT child. The age gap did mean that trying to cope with two children requiring adult supervision didn't last long, which was a relief.

One of the advantages of Jake's ASD, and one feature that really made life easier, was that, other than for entertainment purposes when he was younger, he really didn't pursue social company within the family. He couldn't see the point, thought that socialising was boring and much preferred to be on his own or with a friend playing Xbox or football. This allowed us to give Mollie, a child who craved social interaction and attention, lots of one-on-one attention and time, without feeling guilty that Jake was missing out.

He never appeared to experience or showed any jealousy towards Mollie or the time that she demanded from her parents. As long as he was left to play on his Xbox, he was quite happy and content. Mollie had the majority of the attention within the home and she was always the centre of attention. Ironically, she was very jealous of Jake if she perceived him to be having the tiniest bit of attention. Luckily, for her and for us, this never seemed to bother him.

We tried to ensure that Jake's emotional well-being and development were protected from Mollie by our non-negotiable boundaries. Due to difficulties with friendships, we made a concerted effort to invite boys around to play who also had a specific interest in Xbox and football.

When he had friends round it would drive Mollie up the wall and result in numerous meltdowns that would last for hours. We spent years riding through the storm, providing Jake with his own space and accommodating friends and sleepovers while simultaneously dealing with Mollie's meltdowns.

It was crucial, to us that we preserved this area of his life, especially as it was an area that he needed practice in.

Looking back and with Mollie's input, the reasons for her meltdowns and her continued efforts to sabotage these events have become clearer. She always needs to be the centre of attention and she would be insanely jealous of her brother having friends around and the fact that she was excluded from these interactions. It is worth noting that during these periods we also facilitated play dates for Mollie. This behaviour was not exclusive to the periods of times when she had no friends of her own.

I think that coping with a sibling has been difficult for Mollie. Following a stressful day at school, when she was younger, she would then have to come home and accommodate the needs and wants of another child. It was the same on holidays and so on. In a family of four, she was constantly fighting for attention, trying to control the interactions of everyone, having to accommodate some of the needs of others and trying to avoid the perceived demands of four different people. Even though Jake was happy in his own space playing on his Xbox, allowing him to do this would involve Mollie accommodating this need and allowing it.

Many hours were spent physically removing her from his room. Hours of meltdowns would inevitably ensue and ultimately result in the house being trashed. Although we never backed down on our non-negotiable boundaries, it was approximately three years before these incidents stopped happening. Her desire to control her brother and whatever he is doing still occasionally arises but fortunately Mollie's blow-ups are shorter and much less explosive.

It's hardly surprising that she used to ask me to leave her dad so that it was just us girls together. We just couldn't adequately meet her extreme needs and provide her with the control that she needed until Jake became older and more independent.

How we try to accommodate the needs of both children within the family unit

In the interests of all family members, we often operated as two different families rather than trying to do activities as a unit. I primarily looked after Mollie doing the things that she enjoyed and Lee spent quality time with Jake at football. Jake has been playing football from the age of six and Lee has always either managed or coached his teams. They also went to watch their beloved Stoke City FC together.

Maintaining Jake's interest in football was crucial for us because of the huge positives that came with it. Through football he learned how to socialise better within a group. The team provided a ready-made pool of boys with a similar interest to Jake who could potentially be friends. There was also a useful social side to the football team involving numerous outings and occasions.

By hook and by crook we developed ways to help him control his emotional regulation in order to reduce the extreme outbursts that he had on the pitch. Through football he learned about being part of a team and working with others for the greater good.

Lee managing the team was crucial for Jake to be able to maintain a position. I don't think that his character would, at that time, have been understood and therefore tolerated by another team. Fortunately, the problems that Jake has with his motor skills are limited to his fine motor skills and do not affect his football. He has a real talent and natural flair for football, which has also helped him with his confidence and low self-esteem.

Jake still plays football and he has now moved on to the next level. He now has a new manager but Lee is still very much involved and is the assistant manager and coach. Jake can still struggle with football due to confidence issues that he has when his performance is, in his eyes, less than perfect and the incredibly high standards that he places on himself. He can still have mini meltdowns on the pitch due to frustration but, all in all, maintaining this has been crucial for his development.

I didn't do the practical boy things with Jake due to my responsibilities with Mollie but I became, as Mollie terms it, the sensitive parent. My role with Jake was to understand him and to get to the bottom of emotional issues and provide practical solutions. We have always enjoyed watching films together and even now 9.00pm is our time to watch a film or an episode or two of *Criminal Minds* on Netflix.

As Mollie grew older, her dad's talents became more appealing to her, especially his skills on computers and playing computer games. Now that Jake is older, he really does not want to be doing much with his parents because friends and girls are much more appealing. Lee and I can now take Mollie out together as a family unit of three, because we no longer need to be with one child each. Jake growing up and maturing has definitely helped us to accommodate more fully Mollie's needs and for those needs to be split between two parents. This shift in our family dynamic is quite possibly a contributing factor to the improvements and the easier life that we now experience with her.

Over the years, Lee and I have slotted into specific parenting roles. Lee is the fun guy, the childish one who the kids seem to have more fun with. He is also the practical fixer of things, strong in a crisis and brilliant at anything technical. I am the fixer of emotional issues, the one that the kids come to if they need to talk or get something off their chests. I'm the soft one who they can cuddle up with and watch a film or the TV. I hope I provide the relaxation, sensitivity and calmness to complement the pleasure that they receive from Lee's hyperactive, excitable, fun and practical nature.

20

How Living with PDA Affected My Own Mental Health

One area that is grossly underestimated is the devastating effect that living with a child with PDA can have on the primary caregivers. Parents who are on their knees, running on empty and perhaps, as I was, experiencing very real suicidal thoughts are simply and all too often deemed to be weak and the primary cause of their own problems. Their child, due to not having any clear physical disabilities, may be deemed not disabled enough to require support.

If nothing else, I hope that writing this book and sharing my personal journey with others may help to actually highlight just how complex and challenging living with someone with a hidden disability is. Many families are, as we were, often in crisis and are desperately in need of support from their local services. I did manage to get support and I have a wonderful, supportive family but unfortunately many others don't and are left trying to cope completely on their own.

I would urge any parent or carer whose own mental health is becoming increasingly compromised by caring for an individual with PDA to consult their GP. I found that a small dose of fluoxetine has been greatly beneficial in keeping my nerves and my own mental health far more stable and on an even keel. I also referred myself to Mind, a charity that helps people with mental health issues. I received excellent support and understanding from Mind, and my counsellor was hugely supportive and helpful. Sometimes just having someone who you can offload to without fear of judgement can be hugely beneficial.

In order to illustrate the effects that caring for an individual with PDA can have on the carer, I thought that I would share a couple of my blog posts with you, which were written at the actual time of such feelings. These were not even written during my darkest of hours; I have, at times, felt far worse than even these posts can illustrate.

They may sound self-pitying but this really is how low, isolated and desperate parents may feel. Through my involvement with support groups I know that I am not alone in these thoughts and feelings.

FEELING LOW AND THE EMOTIONAL COST OF BEING A CARER

I wrote this towards the end of Mollie's final school placement during one of my very low spells. I still feel like this sometimes, but I do think that these feelings are something that I have successfully worked through.

Living with Mollie is like swimming in the ocean during a storm. You have to battle every minute of every day just to keep your head above water. You often feel as if you are drowning and when you do manage to come up for air there is always another huge wave, choppy seas and torrential rain to ensure that you are pushed beneath the water yet again. The hardest part is that you know that you will never again experience the pleasure and the calm of dry land because, no matter how hard or how long you swim, the battle with the sea will go on forever and ever.

It is one of these lows that I am feeling today. I have felt it creeping on for the last few days and gradually growing and spreading until I find myself teetering on the edge of mental stability and well-being. I have spent all night crying and I have found myself bursting into tears all morning. These feelings are usually the warning signs that I could be about to enter a bout of depression.

I used to be a powerhouse of strength who could take on the world and relished the challenge of everything that life could throw at me. Sometimes I still feel like that but alternating between feeling strong enough to take on the world and then just wanting to curl up in a corner and disappear – two states of mind that are constantly in conflict with each other.

It is the years of doing battle with the LEA, health professionals, persistent school refusal leading to long periods at home and the ignorance of short-sighted people, combined with simultaneously living in the grips of PDA, that have not only emptied my mental, emotional and physical bank account but have plummeted them into the red.

When your mental and physical reserves are so depleted it gets harder and harder to build them up again and the continual pressure of the life that you lead means that you have to make regular withdrawals. It is a difficult account balance to keep in the black and as the years pass by it becomes harder and harder.

There are many intertwining threads of thoughts and feelings as well as the reality of my daily life that all combine together to bring me down to my knees during one of my lows.

Although I deeply love my daughter and know that she cannot help having PDA, it is an extremely difficult condition to live with and I often feel that I am living in an abusive relationship. My child orders me around, shouts at me, is verbally abusive to me, makes me wait on her hand and foot and calls me horrible names. She has imprisoned me within my home and if I don't comply she can become extremely violent and, through no fault of her own, have very explosive and destructive meltdowns.

I am the adult and she is the child, and I do find the reversal of our status within that relationship and the way that she often treats me totally degrading and it has seriously damaged my self-esteem. There is no alternative because you can't reason, negotiate or change how things are with a child with PDA; you just have to manage it as successfully as possible.

To be isolated in your own home in an abusive relationship with a child who requires constant attention and appears to have the brain of a five-year-old, despite her high IQ and outwardly more normal persona is horrendous and drains the life out of you. It is boring, lonely, isolating, depressing, anxiety-provoking and claustrophobic. You wake up in a morning with just another day of hell to look forward to and each day it gets harder and harder to do.

The rest of the world is just something that surrounds you but that you are no longer a part of. People busy to and fro, work, evenings out, days out, holidays, new relationships, new friends, chitter-chatter, and I view it all from within my bubble. I envy them their normal lives and find it impossible to empathise with their normal day-to-day worries and hassles.

I mourn the loss of my normal life – the one that I had before PDA took over – and I feel that my future life is just a black void of emptiness that stretches out before me. The fact that this reality is for the rest of my life and is not a passing phase or something that will rectify itself is sometimes just too much to bear.

I also mourn the loss of my daughter – the one who I thought I had before PDA consumed her. The child who smiles back at me from early photographs with a cheeky grin and a sparkle in her eyes. I have accepted and love my daughter, PDA or not, but I can't help but cry when I look at those pictures and my heart aches with the loss of what should have been.

I have to be continually in role play and present a persona of myself that just isn't me in order to try and keep Mollie calm and her anxieties low. This is so draining to keep up day after day and I can only manage it for short spurts before the normal me comes back out. The irony of this is that Mollie also has to do this with me. She has to role play the persona of a sweet little girl to try and keep me calm but she can only manage it for short spurts until the real anxiety-ridden Mollie re-emerges.

When one of us drops our role play persona, it has a domino effect, quickly causing the other one to become anxious and drop theirs and the result is 'FIREWORKS'. When this happens I find it increasingly difficult to continue to adopt the strategies and to have the patience to care for Mollie in the way that she needs to keep her self-esteem and emotional well-being intact.

This is my life day in, day out, and it is just the same for my husband. Sometimes I cope well and I parent her to PDA perfection and other times I just spiral into depression, so I have started to look for my triggers. What has caused this quick decline when only a week ago I was on a high, writing my blog, campaigning for the recognition of PDA, enjoying a few but rare successful days out. I felt that my life had a purpose again and that purpose was to use my experiences to help others like me. My life wasn't over, it finally had meaning again; so what has gone wrong?

I am finding the daily trudge of being stuck at home with Mollie just too much to cope with day in, day out. This is a cumulative effect that has been brought on by the reoccurring episodes of school refusal and not because it is the Easter holidays. During the past three years she has only accessed about 17 months of schooling and these have been intermittent rather than in one block, with school holidays to contend with also. We had two weeks of school refusal before the holidays and I face more school refusal after the holidays. My ability to cope with her persistent school refusal is much depleted. Whilst Lee's life is every bit as difficult and as limited as mine, he does have the escape of work and his last remaining hobby, football, whilst I am Mollie's main carer.

My blog and my desire to spread awareness of PDA have given me something really good to focus on. I have never used the world of social media before and I even opened Facebook and Twitter accounts to spread the word. Then last night I had, for no apparent reason, my Twitter account suspended. This tiny blip has really upset me because one of the few things that I was enjoying and that had given me a sense of purpose has been taken away from me and is beyond my control. When you are already starting to struggle, little things going wrong can become magnified in your mind and you lose all sense of perspective.

Also, the complete lack of any control that I have over my own life means that I cannot cope when a tiny morsel of control that I have managed to acquire is taken away from me. Like Mollie, I now have very little tolerance for any control being exerted over by others. Or for any of my last remaining bastions of control to be removed from me by anyone or anything. Mollie has simply emptied my tolerance-to-demands tank and drunk it dry.

Opening a Facebook account has been wonderful in many ways and it has opened up a much-needed link to the outside world. I was browsing through the pages of people who I haven't seen for 26 years and I stumbled on a few old school pictures and all the emotions of seeing myself as a young teenager just took over. I have no sentiment for school – I hated it – but at least in those photos I had youth on my side and the whole world at my feet.

My future stretched out before me in a world that held so many promises. I looked at that picture and I burst into tears and I am crying as I write this blog. I felt sorry for that girl in the picture because she looked so happy and had no idea of what life had in store for her. When I look at that picture I don't see *me* anymore because I feel as if that life belonged to a different person.

I know that I have a lot in life to be grateful for and that there are many people who are in a far more desperate position than I. I often tell myself this when I am low to give myself a good old kick up the backside and just get on with it. However, if I am writing a blog I need to be honest with the people who are good enough to read it and today this is how I feel. Perhaps tomorrow I will feel differently or perhaps this is the start of a gradual slide that I will just have to endure and wait to come out of on the other side.

I must emphasise that I do receive excellent support from my parents who are phoning me daily and practically begging to have Mollie for me. In the past, I have just carried on, regardless of how bad things have got but then you do run the risk of a complete breakdown and an inability to provide Mollie with the care and support that she needs.

My support network know that they have to keep me strong during these times so that I can quickly recover and resume my normal duties. My husband has taken half a day off work to give me a complete break from Mollie, which will, I hope, do the job. I will keep my parents for emergency use only as I am painfully aware of how fragile their own physical and mental health is.

Mollie is so complex and challenging that looking after her does require a group effort. Even with that group effort, it is impossible for me, as the main carer, to cope with her without the occasional injection of added support, which I am fortunate enough to have. How parents cope without a partner or the support of a good family I really do not know and I am filled with admiration for those who do.

HAS MY ENVIRONMENT ALTERED MY BRAIN?

The following blog post was written to try and explain how much my own brain and my ability to cope seemed to have altered as a result of living with PDA. I do wonder if living under extreme circumstances does produce permanent changes in the chemical makeup of the brain.

During the past few years, Mollie and I have found ourselves on an incredible journey. It has been tough, upsetting, debilitating, exasperating, frustrating and exhausting. I have found myself precariously wobbling on the edge of mental stability for the majority of the journey and desperately clinging on to avoid falling into the huge black void time and time again. Fight or flight is now a permanent mental state that continually hangs around my neck like a noose.

I feel that the environment that I have been exposed to during the past ten years with Mollie layered on top of 14 difficult years with Jake (Asperger's) and 20 stressful years with my husband (Asperger's and OCD, although he has been much better during the last three years) have permanently altered my own personality and ability to cope with life.

Here is a short description of me in the years prior to the years of extreme stress. I was a very confident, outgoing and social person. Nothing fazed me and I relished every challenge that life could throw at me. Nothing could overload me. If it needed to be done I would get it done; what others couldn't manage I would happily put on my to-do list. You could place a mountain in front of me and I would simply jump over it; climbing wasn't required.

I ran a business and helped to set up a large, bed retail business whilst simultaneously balancing a hectic home life with a husband who was always mentally ill, a son who was challenging and difficult and a daughter who was delightful but also extremely challenging. I coped; I did it all; I was the lynchpin of the family – the one who kept everything going. I was mum, wife, cleaner, cook, psychiatrist and behaviour analyst for my family, advocate for all of their needs and a successful businesswoman. A powerhouse of strength and determination coupled with a belief that I could and I would do whatever I set my mind to and no one, but no one, could stop me.

Boy was I about to learn a tough lesson in life: I was not invincible; I was but a mere mortal! When I did crash it was with the force of a nuclear explosion and I will never recover. It would appear that the years of coping were simply laying the foundations for the impeding explosion. Little by little the anxiety caused by the stress of coping was building and building until it could stay inside no longer. My brain could not absorb anymore anxiety or stress and my cortisol levels had reached maximum. Fight or flight was, by now, a permanent state of mind.

Eventually when my brain could cope and absorb no longer – BOOM!!!! I felt as if a nuclear bomb has exploded in my head, leaving certain areas destroyed and, while other areas were still working, they could soon shut down and needed to recuperate. Other areas appeared to have received gamma rays and turned my brain into a green hulk of an intellectual sponge that had an insatiable thirst for information. So what did actually create this penultimate crash and spectacular fall to Earth?

Perhaps it was the year in, year out bombardment of stress and anxiety that I had barely noticed because I always thought that I could cope. I had setbacks along the years but I would always bounce back even stronger, or so I thought. This was coupled with the huge amount of stress and frustration that comes with having a child whose behaviour is so challenging, so extreme and so misunderstood that it is incorrectly attributed to other causes, namely my parenting skills, by professionals.

The years of begging to be listened to and having door after door shut in my face when I tried to reach out to CAMHS to get the correct help for both of my children was bound to take its toll and was so difficult to deal with emotionally. As each door shut I became increasingly disheartened – alone – I felt disrespected by others and unfairly judged.

The years of listening to unhelpful and quite frankly downright stupid and insensitive remarks from the ignorant. Why do these people, who have no experience of challenging behaviour, always think that they are so damn wonderful at all aspects of child rearing? Why do they feel that they have the right to judge those who do have this first-hand experience? Why do they wrongly assume that I want to hear their pointless advice or have any interest in being told, 'Give her to me for a week, I'd soon sort her out, she'd soon learn with me.' Really, how I would love to see them try!

I can only describe living with Mollie between the ages of five and nine as hell on earth. This was an abusive relationship that stripped away every ounce of my confidence and emotional well-being.

The intrusion into one's life does eventually become unbearable to cope with especially when there are multiple agencies involved. The involvement is necessary to access the support but baring your soul in attempts to beg for help and understanding is a humiliating experience to go through.

This is me now, post-breakdown.

I have withdrawn from society because, if the truth be known, I don't really like people anymore. People make me anxious and nervous, they judge, criticise, comment on things that they know nothing about, show my greater knowledge on this topic no respect, undermine me and pull me down. There are, of course, exceptions to this and I do have a very close inner circle of people who do not fall into this category.

I need calm, peace and tranquillity and when I don't get this in my environment I can soon go into sensory overload. Even noise in the house can get the old heart racing and the anxiety rising. I can't stand noise! My once-fabulous short-term memory, multitasking and organising skills are now pretty much defunct. Remembering birthdays, or not as the case may be, is an increasing cause of stress and anxiety especially when I do forget one. I can only concentrate on one thing at a time without going into panic mode and too many people bustling around me when I am trying to concentrate and organise quickly sends me into a state of panic.

My thought processes have become rigid, and a sudden change of plan can and does send me into a tailspin. Life has to be in order and I need to know what to expect so that I can mentally prepare myself. Going with the flow is not an option at the moment. The easiest way for me to keep myself calm and reduce anxiety is to spend most of my time at home, which, by the way, I am more than happy to do – this isn't a negative thing. Being a social butterfly is only a positive if you derive positive experiences from it; I derive much more positive and fulfilling experiences from being either on my own or with my nearest and dearest.

Whilst my short-term memory appears to have gone AWOL, my ability to learn about things that I am interested in and retain that information has gone through the roof. I am like a computer that requires constant input but within a relatively narrow field of topics. PDA, autism and anything that can help me understand my children more, are top of that list.

My environment has caused me such high levels of stress and anxiety that, I feel, my brain has been permanently altered. This doesn't mean that it is a negative thing or something to mourn; I am quite happy and at peace with my new self.

Who says I need to be socialising in order to be a productive and important member of society or to be happy and fulfilled. My pleasure and fulfilment simply come from different areas now, which does not mean that I am any less; I am just different to how I used to be. I was a caterpillar, but now I am a butterfly. I have simply gone through a process of metamorphosis.

21

Supporting a Family Living with PDA

I wholeheartedly believe, in fact I know, that without my wonderful support network I would not have been able to implement or maintain the lifestyle changes that are essential for Mollie's progress. An adequate support package is essential for the best prognosis, both for the family as a whole and the individual with PDA.

Words can never accurately describe just how stressful, exhausting, isolating, upsetting and nerve shattering living with PDA can be for the individual with PDA and for the family supporting him/her. Because, at times, everything can be so hard and appear so bleak, you really can lose all sight of any of the positives. With the correct support, it has been possible for us to strike a more harmonious balance between the positive and negative experiences. The restoration of this balance was and still is crucial for the long-term prognosis of our family.

PDA is not currently included in any of the official diagnostic manuals, so parents really can be left up the creek without a paddle, which only adds to the huge mountain that we already have to climb.

In addition to the huge struggles that parents may face when rearing a child with PDA, we also have to deal with the ignorance that comes from family, friends and professionals who simply will not acknowledge that such a condition can possibly exist let alone understand it. Instead of receiving help and support, many parents may find that they are judged, ridiculed and unfairly blamed for producing a wilful and challenging child, at their own hand, by ineffective and weak parenting.

As long as professionals hold the parents accountable and view the child as NT, but with behavioural and emotional issues, rather than actually having a diagnosable developmental disorder, then any support offered will be few and far between if not non-existent.

This view, which is shared by many professionals who have usually done no actual research into PDA, is a major stumbling block and may prevent the process of an assessment for ASD, support within the school, respite for the parents and the understanding of family and friends. It can strip parents of the very support that is crucial for survival.

I have been extremely lucky and I have a lot of support from my family, social services and, in the past, education services. Have you noticed the one, and possibly the most crucial, service that has offered us no support at all with regard to PDA, until recently? Yes, you've guessed it, *health*!

Because PDA is not recognised, understood or diagnosed in my local area, I have received no support in how to cope or manage my child from my local health services. Like many parents, we have had to research, learn and develop a successful framework of strategies without any professional input whatsoever.

We were well and truly left high and dry, not to mention alone, to navigate our way through life with PDA with no map, no compass and no supplies. Until professionals decide to research and educate themselves on PDA and the successful handling strategies, increasing numbers of parents, children and adults with PDA will continue to remain unsupported and failed by the system.

My support network

A solid marriage and supportive husband have been crucial for me, not just from the point of view of sharing the load of Mollie, but also because of the emotional support that we have had to offer each other during our many battles with the authorities.

My husband and I have been together for 23 years and although it hasn't always been plain sailing, we now work as a partnership for Mollie. It is so important that both partners are pulling in the right direction and singing from the same hymn sheet. How single parents cope I do not know and this only further emphasises the urgent support that parents do need. If you are a single-parent family, my admiration and my heart go out to you.

I am lucky enough to have the most wonderful and supportive parents who have fully taken on-board PDA and the recommended strategies. Initially it wasn't easy for them to fully understand PDA but they listened, learned and educated themselves. They have a very strong and loving relationship with Mollie even though they have also been victims of her violent and verbal abuse.

They learnt, no matter how upsetting it was for them, to ignore, move on and, most importantly, to understand why she was exhibiting such extreme and challenging behaviour. I think that they learned and did what they did out of love and a desire, regardless of what was asked of them, to support me and my husband.

I know that both of my parents have been deeply troubled and upset by the emotional wreck that they have often seen me reduced to. I am, after all, still their little girl, no matter how old or wrinkled I get. They were willing to do whatever it took in order to help me as much as they could. This included missing holidays and often having to offer me daily support during my periods of complete breakdown. Their unwavering support continues to this day.

My outreach team took the time and effort to read about PDA when I suggested it to them and they became wonderful advocates for Mollie and PDA within social services. Their willingness to learn about PDA meant that they immediately recognised how much Mollie fitted that profile.

They abandoned the traditional behaviour strategies that they had tried, which had failed with Mollie, and adopted the recommended PDA ones instead. They quickly saw that these strategies produced more positive results and wholeheartedly promoted them and educated others within social services about PDA.

It was because of their testaments explaining how complex and challenging that Mollie was, given during my many review meetings and battles with their superiors, that I finally won a package of support that actually met my needs. During our toughest times I managed to negotiate three hours of outreach a week alongside seven hours of direct payments a week so that I could employ someone to help me with Mollie. I no longer receive the outreach, due to Mollie refusing to engage, but I do still receive the seven hours of direct payments.

Mollie's wonderful educational psychologist, Eric, who sadly passed away in 2013, was extremely well respected within education services. By chance, he had been trained by Professor Elizabeth Newson alongside Phil Christie, so he was fully on-board with PDA and was the first professional that suggested it to me. His influence within education services definitely helped us to gain the correct support, understanding and strategies. He had a love, a desire and a passion for his work and for the families and the children who he helped. He was still working extremely long hours well into his seventies, when he passed away from a sudden and unexpected illness.

Ann is Mollie's personal assistant who provides seven hours of respite a week funded by direct payments. She has known Mollie since she was a baby, and she is brilliant. She plays with Mollie on her level, offers her friendship and companionship and supports me. She has never questioned or judged our choices, lifestyle or strategies and she took on the concept of PDA fully from the outset. She has formed a strong bond with Mollie, which goes beyond the seven hours of paid support that she provides.

An online support network via forums and social media were my lifeline when it came to those early days of understanding and getting to grips with PDA. It was here that I received the best advice possible and support from those who walk in my shoes. I have also met and made some wonderful friends through these support networks. When you are living with PDA it is easy to become disconnected with the NT world and you can begin to lose the connections that you have previously enjoyed with friends. You may no longer feel a part of their world and similarly they may find it difficult to understand or empathise with your current situation. Within the support groups we can find friends who have the shared interest of PDA.

Even with the fantastic support that I have had and the lucky breaks within some services that enabled greater understanding, it is important not to underestimate the huge amount of work and research that I also put into defending my own case and demanding the correct amount of support. I really do think that those who shout the loudest will eventually get the most.

Mollie is, I believe, at the most extreme end of the PDA spectrum and she has spent the best part of the past four years at home on a full-time basis. Even with the support of my family, I would not have coped and would continue to struggle now without the additional support that the seven hours of respite offers me.

It is important to remember that Mollie rarely leaves the home, so many tasks that other families simply take for granted, like going to the shop or collecting a prescription, simply can't be carried out. Most of the seven hours is spent simply doing run-of-the-mill chores that I can only do when I have cover for Mollie.

I consider myself to be a pretty strong and resourceful person, so I cannot help but wonder how families with no support – sometimes single parents – manage to survive, let alone adequately support their child. I know that these wonderful parents do exist because I see them on support groups but I really do not know how they continue to function. Their mental and physical strength must know no bounds; during times when I am feeling a little bit sorry for myself I always remember the single parents with no support to remind me of how lucky I am.

I cannot express enough how desperate and how thoroughly deserving a family living with PDA are when it comes to the need for a strong and effective support network. For many families, support is not a luxury to enable a parent to have a few hours of being pampered; it is a necessity for the long-term survival of the family unit. It enables the parent to have sufficient help so that they can continue to offer the incredibly high levels of support that individuals with PDA often require.

Top tips for supporting a family living with PDA

The first and the most important tip, whether you are a professional, friend or a family member, is that you have to educate yourself and really take on board the concept of PDA. How can you support a family if you don't understand the condition and the manner in which the individual with PDA requires managing? You need to be open to the idea from the start; trying to convince someone who is there to support you that PDA does exist is draining and time wasting.

Offer as much support as you can, especially if you are a professional. I understand that funds are increasingly tight and the number of families requiring support is rising, however the mental flexibility and strength required to support an individual with PDA, combined with often coping with daily abuse, can crush the strongest of us. Please do not underestimate the needs of these families, especially single-parent families and families without the support of extended family or friends.

Do not suggest traditional behaviour management strategies, reward charts, being firm or anything along those lines to a family living with PDA. We have already been there, got the T-shirt and the film. Whether you are a professional or family member, please respect our knowledge about PDA, our child and their unique needs.

We have often, through trial and error and years of hands-on experience, become the experts within this field. There is nothing as tiring, frustrating or degrading as repeatedly having to justify our life choices to those who have no experience of walking in our shoes. Please trust, respect and bow to our greater knowledge when it comes to supporting us with our child. We've been doing it for years, we have learnt the hard way and we have to pay the price when those who are less experienced make crucial mistakes because they think that they know best.

The most dependable, reliable and useful source of support can come from our families. This isn't always possible, but if you are supporting a family member living with PDA please offer them as much support as you can while refraining from any judgemental remarks. You will undoubtedly become the most important link in their support network.

Part 8

Diagnosis

22

Why Recognition and Diagnosis are So Important

I, as do many other parents and professionals, feel that it is absolutely essential that PDA is officially recognised, diagnosed and classified as a separate syndrome within the autism spectrum.

PDA is now being diagnosed and recognised in increasing numbers by clinicians, local authorities, social services and schools. In just a few short years, awareness and information about PDA on the internet has mushroomed, and the annual PDA conferences are usually oversubscribed.

Although the PDA movement is moving in the correct direction, it is still painfully slow for those parents who are living in areas where PDA is not recognised. Getting a diagnosis and appropriate support for your child with PDA is very much a postcode lottery depending on your local authority.

There is huge debate among professionals as to the validity of PDA as a separate and stand-alone diagnosis. As far as I am aware this debate isn't about whether a group of children with this profile exist but it is instead about whether this group of children requires a separate diagnosis of PDA or the existing labels in the diagnostic manual are already sufficient to cover them.

Many children who fit the PDA profile have had no specific diagnoses or they have had alternative diagnoses (such as Asperger's syndrome, oppositional defiance disorder, attachment disorder or ADHD) that don't fully describe or make sense of their complete profile and the accompanying guidelines for intervention aren't effective. This can be confusing and frustrating for parents.

Using PDA as a separate diagnosis within the autism spectrum puts these children into a collective group with the correct profile, understanding, strategies, label and signpost for others to follow. As discussed by Christie *et al.* 2011 the true purpose of the correct diagnosis is so that others can collectively better understand the child's behaviours:

> It is often said of children with PDA that they are 'complex'; and while this is certainly true, it also reflects the fact that they confuse people and that there is variation in the way that different people understand them and their behaviour. A diagnosis should be about reaching a shared understanding of a child's profile; a formulation that can lead to an agreed way of making sense of his behaviour. (Christie *et al.* 2011, p.34)

The benefits of a diagnosis of PDA for children and adults

A diagnosis of PDA immediately signposts parents, the individuals with PDA and caregivers to the correct support, strategies and support groups. An individual with PDA can then research the literature available so that they can better understand their own life and needs. Parents and carers can use the information to help them better understand and to care for their child or the individual who they are supporting.

Failure to diagnose individuals with PDA means that they may never be given the opportunity to fully understand themselves, be truly understood by others, have access to the correct support and strategies or be given the chance to achieve and be the best that they can possibly be. Because the most successful handling strategies are unique to PDA, it is crucial for an individual to be correctly diagnosed so that they can access these strategies.

Additionally, failure to recognise PDA can lead to an incorrect diagnosis that neither adequately describes the individual and his/her difficulties nor provides the correct strategies, for example strategies that are usually successful for individuals with ASD or conduct problems do not tend to be successful for individuals with PDA.

Many clinicians don't believe in diagnosing or 'labelling' at all. Instead, they believe in looking at the individual as a whole, rather than as a condition, and feel that providing the correct strategies for the individual is the best way forward. I really do not understand this ethos at all. Why waste valuable time trying to find the best strategies for an individual when a diagnosis gives you a fast-track signpost to the recommended strategies, which can then be tailored to the individual person?

A set of strategies does not give the parents, caregivers or the individual concerned any understanding of the underlying condition or the difficulties that are driving the behaviour. Strategies can make so much more sense if we understand why we need to use them.

A diagnosis endures over time and will provide understanding, strategies and an immediate signpost for the individual for life. A set of strategies without a diagnosis does not, and professionals who come into

260 Pathological Demand Avoidance Syndrome – My Daughter is Not Naughty

contact with the individual in the future may attempt to make their own diagnosis. They may disagree with previous successful strategies and insist on a return to more traditional strategies in the belief that tried and tested behavioural support has to be the way forward. For the individual with PDA this would be disastrous!

An accurate diagnosis of a physical ailment is crucial for the correct understanding and treatment plan. If a person is physically ill, it is deemed normal for an individual and their family to want to know what the problem is, for a diagnosis to be made and for a relevant treatment that is successful for that illness to be administered.

When an individual has a neurological condition, people only want to be shown the same courtesy and respect. We are not trying to label our loved one for the sake of it. We simply want their neurological condition to be specifically identified so that we can offer the best psychological intervention possible.

A diagnosis is essential in order to access many services and support, for example in my experience, social service's outreach service will not support families if the individual does not have a diagnosis. A diagnosis is essential for children who are still accessing education to receive the correct support and approach from staff in the school setting. Again, I'm baffled by the ethos of CAMHS, in some areas, to not assess and diagnose first and foremost.

23

Navigating the Bumpy and Winding Road to Diagnosis

Persuading any professional that your child is not developing or behaving in a typical manner for a child of his/her age is always difficult. The initial reaction is that you are worrying over nothing, that you just need to stop comparing your child with other children, perhaps you need to be stricter, or that he/she will grow out of it and so on.

So what is the best way to proceed if you think that your child may have PDA? How do you get anyone to believe you or to take you seriously when all that the outside world can see is a child who can, at times, appear to be typical of other children both in behaviour and presentation? How do you manage to convey the immense struggles at home when everything can appear to be so calm in other settings?

Alternatively, you may have a child who can be very charming and social as well as explosive and challenging, both at school and at home. This solves one problem, from the point of view that the behaviour can be seen across two settings. However, good eye contact and surface sociability may mean that ASD is discounted straight away, often leading to a less suitable conclusion of poor parenting, oppositional defiance disorder or attachment disorder as the root cause of your child's difficulties.

Using my experiences of what approaches and methods have worked for me, as well as with those that have failed, I thought that I would share a plan of action that may be helpful on your path to diagnosis. I cannot guarantee that this plan will bring you any joy or that it will ultimately secure you a diagnosis, but it may be a good framework within which to begin.

One of the most important things that I have learned is that some, but not all professionals do not like a parent telling them what the problem is. A well-read, well-researched and articulate parent can be seen as a 'nuisance, arrogant, know it all' at best or a 'Dr Internet', 'label obsessive', 'Münchausen by proxy candidate' at worse.

Looking back at my own experiences, the services that did come to accept PDA and treat me as an equal were social services and education services. I can only assume that these relationships were built on mutual respect as we worked and collaborated together to try and discover, solve and 'wrongly' discipline the behaviour out of Mollie.

This happened because I was ignorant about ASD and PDA. I was willing to follow their lead and became gradually more assertive over time. We discovered together that nothing worked and agreed together that PDA made perfect sense for her behaviours. Strong relationships and mutual respect were built during this time, which continued to serve us all well.

By the time it came to asserting myself with the medical professionals, I was extremely well-read and self-educated on Asperger's and PDA. I was horrified to realise that my own knowledge had now surpassed many of the very professionals on whom I was relying to teach me. I do not think that this was well received, and vocalising my shock at their apparent lack of knowledge did nothing to help my cause. Following a few disputes, the medical ranks closed around me and I was essentially blackballed from my local mental health services for two years.

What I learned from this experience is that it is imperative for parents to tread very carefully and very respectfully, even if we don't feel like it, in order to receive the best understanding and support for your child.

Step one: Make a case to support your claims

First, write a timeline of your child's development and behaviour from birth until the present day. Try to make it as relevant and as to the point as possible. Note developmental milestones, like walking, babbling and talking, as well as challenging or confusing behaviours and the period in your child's development when these began and ended.

If it is possible, ask for someone else to support your description of your child. A short report from a teacher would be ideal, however if your child flies under the radar at school a short report from a family member, friend or the leader of an extra curricula activity would still be useful.

The important thing is to try to emphasise that the difficulties that are arising are not just witnessed by you and that they occur in two different settings. If your child does show challenging behaviour in school, you may already be in the fortunate position of having an array of observation sheets and reports that you can include in your file.

Next, print some information from the internet detailing PDA, which can be used to compare to your child's timeline. The PDA Society website[3] has a diagnostic criteria page, which may be useful. There is also an abundance of information on PDA collected from all over the internet. It would be useful to highlight why you feel that your child fits this diagnostic criteria by providing written examples of how his/her own behaviours mirror those described in the official descriptions.

A parent screening questionnaire, the EDA-Q, is also available and can be downloaded from the PDA Society website or from The PDA Resource website. This is an easy and simple questionnaire to complete and score. The score will indicate the likelihood of whether an individual may have PDA.

It would also be useful to make a comprehensive list of all of your child's personality traits, like I have done for Mollie in the appendices of the book. This enables clinicians to see that your child's difficulties are in line with the difficulties associated with ASD. This can help them to understand all areas of difficulty for your child with greater insight than simply focusing on challenging behaviour, which is more often than not put down to parenting.

If your child does fly under the radar at school it may be useful to print some evidence supporting this fact. There is considerable literature on the internet by experienced professionals within the field of autism who describe how some children can hold in behaviours in the day at the expense of being far worse at home for their parents.

Step two: Visit the doctor

Share your concerns about your child's development with your GP and explain that you would greatly appreciate

---

3   The PDA Society website is available at www.pdasociety.org.uk.

a referral to CAMHS. There may not be any need to produce your evidence at this stage. GPs are often the gateway to other services, so as long as you can express genuine reasons and concerns about your child's complex and challenging needs, you should be able to secure an appointment at CAMHS.

It is better to request or appeal than to demand. Getting from my GP to a CAMHS appointment is not something that I have found problematic in the past and so I hope you won't either.

Step three: Child and Adolescent Mental Health Services (CAMHS)

Either prior to arriving at CAMHS or following your first appointment you may be required to attend the obligatory parenting course. Unfortunately, this is one of the hoops that you may need to jump through in order to progress to the next level. I knew that it would be pointless and time wasting for us, but we still went through the process so that we could advance to the next level.

You may wish to inform your contact at CAMHS that you have written a timeline of your child's development and have made a full profile of their personality traits and areas of difficulty and leave it with him/her along with any other reports from school, reports from family and so on.

It may be wise to attend a few appointments, which allows you to share more details of your difficulties and to bounce ideas off each other, before mentioning PDA. It is important to appear to be problem solving and working together at this stage. A good relationship between you and your contact at CAMHS may be vital for your case, both now and in the future. Patience at this stage may actually save you time and speed the process up in the long run.

Following a few appointments, or when you feel that the time is right, you could bring up the subject of PDA. You could explain that you were searching the internet in an effort to educate yourself on challenging behaviour when you stumbled across a condition that appears to fit your child like a glove. If your child does fly under the radar at school, it may be prudent to point out to your contact at CAMHS that this is one of the features of some children with PDA. You could also ask your child's teacher to look for whether your child is exhibiting any of the more subtle features of avoidance, for example not performing academically in line with the school's expectations given his/her intellect.

You could explain that you have printed the relevant information and made notes on how your child appears to fit these criteria and ask if they mind having a look at this profile in conjunction with the knowledge that they already have about your child. You may point out that you do understand that this condition is a contentious diagnosis that is not widely recognised or in a diagnostic manual but that you would value their opinion all the same. It is always advisable to leave information with professionals so that they can read and digest information at their leisure rather than in a hurry during an appointment.

If attachment disorder or oppositional defiant disorder are suggested as possible reasons for your child's behaviours, you can use the information from the frequently-asked-questions section of this book to try to redirect this train of thought. Research has shown that children with PDA do have behavioural overlaps with children with ASD and with children with conduct problems but that they also have unique characteristics that are not seen in either of the other two groups.

Reactive attachment disorder is a behavioural condition and not a neurological condition. This occurs due to extreme neglect during early infancy. This condition should not be diagnosed unless this is consistent with the child's background and the child should also be assessed to ensure that they don't meet the criteria for ASD prior to receiving a diagnosis.

Step four: Referral for diagnosis

It is hoped that your contact at CAMHS will see how the profile fits your child and will be open to trying PDA strategies. At this stage, you may find that the time is right to enquire about whether your local services are aware and have experience of PDA and are prepared to assess children for it. This may be through CAMHS or you may need a referral to an ASD diagnostic team.

A diagnosis of ASD with a PDA profile is ideal because it not only states that your child has PDA but it also highlights that PDA is an ASD. Mollie was assessed at the Elizabeth Newson Centre and the wording that they used was: 'Mollie has an autism spectrum disorder whose profile most closely fits that of PDA'.

If your local services accept that your child does appear to fit the profile of PDA but do not have the experience to assess or diagnose your child, then you could ask that they apply for funding for a referral to the Elizabeth Newson Centre. If your local services agree to assess for PDA I would be tempted to ask what experience they have in this field and what training have they received with regard to recognising and diagnosing PDA.

Some areas may have the experience and be happy to assess but may suggest offering a diagnosis of 'ASD only' because they believe that they are acting in your best interests by not giving you a direct diagnosis of PDA due to it not being widely recognised. In this situation, I would request that the report states that your child has ASD with a profile that closely resembles PDA and that PDA strategies would be of benefit to your child.

Step five: Options if you can't get a referral

If your local services do not believe in labelling, or in PDA, then you may only have a few options left at your disposal.

You can continue to visit CAMHS in the hope that they eventually see the light, take on board the strategies and agree to diagnose or to refer. Try and keep relationships amicable so that you don't burn your bridges with regard to any future support that you may need. It may also be helpful to request a referral to a paediatrician in the hope that they take your concerns seriously, offer their professional opinion to CAMHS and decide that a diagnostic assessment by an experienced clinician is needed.

Alternatively you can ask your GP to refer you for a private assessment, which you will need to pay for yourself. When Mollie was diagnosed the cost was £2600 although this may have increased now. Please take steps to ensure that any private diagnosis will be recognised by your local services. If it is recognised by education services and social services, this may be all you need to ensure the correct support for your child.

You could contact your local MP with details about your case, the lack of appropriate services in your area and why you desperately need funding for an out-of-area assessment. I know several people who have had success with this route of action.

You could even appeal to your local clinical commissioning group directly (This group is now responsible for local services and funding[4]), stating your case and the long-term damage that the incorrect diagnosis and lack of support could have on your child.

You may have to resort to writing to someone of high authority within CAMHS and complaining that, by refusing to acknowledge a condition that is now being more widely recognised and by refusing to refer your child for an out-of-area assessment, they are failing him/her and his/her needs. You could explain that due to the disastrous consequences that this could have for your child, you feel that you have been left with no alternative other than to make an official complaint.

If this doesn't provoke them into action then you could make an official complaint about your NHS services to PALS (Patient Advice and Liaison Service).

Please think very carefully before taking any serious action and be prepared for any potential fallout that you may incur if you make an official complaint.

Referral and diagnosis can be a long and rocky road. I hope that this information may help to guide you and navigate you through your journey. I can't promise you success and you may hit a few brick walls, but I do hope that this chapter at least gives you a starting point and a framework within which to work.

---

4   For more information please see www.england.nhs.uk/wp-content/uploads/2013/03/a-functions-ccgs.pdf.

Part 9

Final Thoughts

24

The Funny and Endearing Side of PDA

There is a lighter side to PDA that I thought I would try to share with you. Although living with PDA is extremely tough and challenging, there are also lots of really funny and endearing moments. Now that Mollie's life and environment are more suited to her needs, we have the joy of experiencing more and more of the 'lighter side of PDA'. This is a phrase coined by another parent when she began her own Facebook group for parents to share the more delightful aspects of PDA with each other. I hope that this chapter makes you smile and helps you to see the positive aspects of these unique, often misunderstood but very wonderful, brave and courageous individuals.

One of the features of PDA speech is that some children can have quite complex language but it can appear odd, as if the words would sound more suitable coming out of an older child's or even an adult's mouth. The comments that trip off Mollie's tongue can make me either cringe with embarrassment or howl with laughter. The same can be said for her body language, facial expressions and mannerisms. In Mollie's case they have always been very over-exaggerated with a mimicking quality that resembles the type of body language used in children's TV sitcoms. Perhaps it is all part and parcel of the role play element of PDA. She is also very in tune with when people are using persuasive measures to try to encourage her to conform or to respond positively to something. After all, it is in this area that she is the 'master' and so she sees straight through it. Here are just a few of Mollie's more comical moments and her amazing powers at detecting the ulterior motives of others.

At the tender age of four, Mollie and I received a home visit from her wonderful educational psychologist, Eric. During the visit Eric tried a little bit of reverse psychology on Mollie. 'I think that you really do like school Mollie and that you will miss not going everyday', commented Eric. 'I hate it everyone bosses me about', was Mollie's response to which Eric replied, 'But what about all of your friends and all of the fun things that you do at school?' At this, Mollie slowly turned her head, looked Eric straight in the eye and said, 'I know what you are doing, you are trying to get me to say that I like school and I'm telling you now that it isn't going to work'. Eric looked at Lee and I and chuckled at Mollie's incredible powers of perception. For now, he had been well and truly outmanoeuvred by a four-year-old. This was the start of a wonderful and supportive relationship for all of us.

The most embarrassing occasions can be when Mollie decides to tell it exactly how it is; this is also something that she can do as a means of control. If she doesn't want a particular person in the house, insulting them can be a quick and efficient way to get rid of them.

We had a phase of staff coming in from Crossroads (now called Carers Trust) for an hour a week and the staff turnaround was quite high meaning that she couldn't really get used to one person. Mollie really didn't want to interact with them; she was about seven years old and this was during her worst period for meltdowns and fear of people that she didn't know. As soon as the doorbell rang she would beat me to it and open the door. The poor soul on the other side would immediately be told, 'You're so old, fat and ugly just go away.' Then she would slam the door shut in their face whilst they stood completely bemused, horrified and shocked on the other side. The word cringe, as I gingerly opened the door to try to smooth things over, just doesn't cover it! To get past first base with Mollie, you had to be young and pretty and if you weren't, well, you could just forget it.

As we passed through the electronic wristband turnstile to get on a ride at Blackpool Pleasure Beach the attendant made a huge and catastrophic error that will probably haunt him for the rest of his days. 'Excuse me,' he said to Mollie, 'would you just go and stand by the height line so that I can check if you are tall enough?' She did a prompt 180-degree turn and, looking like Chucky on speed with a purple face full of rage, she chastised him in front of the whole queue: 'I don't need to have my height checked. I've been on this ride lots and lots of times, I've even been on the "Big One" for God's sake. Do you really think that if I can go on the Big One that I need to check my height for this little ride you silly man?' She was only about eight years old at the time of this incident.

The poor bloke began to stutter and apologised for his error whilst I silently prayed for the ground to open up and swallow me. As the queue moved forward we heard the poor attendant say to another chap in the queue, 'I only asked if I could check her height, I thought she was going to punch me.' At this point Lee and I exchanged a little glance and had a little titter. Of course we did produce our 'autism alert card' (a card that explains that an individual has a neurological condition that causes difficulties and anxiety associated with social interaction and communication), apologise and explain the situation to him. Following which he enjoyed a lot of playful banter with Mollie every time we went back on the ride.

Back to trying to outwit Mollie, and it's over to my wonderful outreach team. During the early days, before any of us really understood Mollie, they desperately wanted to get Mollie out of the house so that they could interact with her alone. They didn't have a problem with me, but Mollie had developed a bit of an attachment issue, which we were trying to address.

On this particular day, it was snowing outside, so we were all very pleased when, following a period of substantial negotiation helped by the novelty of the recent snow, she finally agreed to play with them in the street while I stayed in the house. We should have known better, and our joy was short lived. Within a few short minutes I noticed that Mollie was sat in the lounge looking rather smug. I wondered what fate had befallen the outreach team and I pondered where they could be.

It was then that the doorbell rang and I realised that a rather deflated outreach team had been the latest victims of the master manipulator. She had cunningly led them outside, lulled them into false sense of security, then dashed back in the house, locked them out and plonked herself back down in front of the TV. I must add that a similar fate occurred to quite a few of us – her dad, my dad and I have all fallen victim to being locked out of the house at one point or another.

It wasn't long before a new outreach worker was to face the initiation process of all things PDA. Upon arrival Mollie told him that he was fat and needed to lose some weight. She took him into the garage, where we have our cross-trainer, and proceeded to put him through weight-loss camp.

While he was exercising she insisted on spraying him with water, which he didn't like. He told Mollie that he was not prepared to let her spray him with water and that he would stop exercising if she continued. Mollie, without a fuss or a cross word, stopped spraying him and he patted himself on the back. This PDA wasn't too bad to deal with after all, he thought, he had succeeded where others had failed. Mollie congratulated him on his work out and handed him a towel with which to mop his sweaty brow. He gratefully took the towel and wiped his face, even more amazed at Mollie's helpfulness. It was only when he looked in the mirror a short while later that he realised that he become the latest victim at the hands of the master manipulator. Mollie had skilfully put blue paint on the blue towel and he now saw a very shocked blue face staring back at him in the mirror.

Mollie seemed very keen on a school that I had found and because it was a few miles away she had agreed that it would be a good idea to stay on a residential basis Monday to Friday. During a home visit Eric, her educational psychologist, asked, 'Now Mollie are you sure about this and you won't change your mind? We don't want to sort this out for you if you are going to refuse to go and it will cost such a lot of money.' At this point Mollie cut him short, looked directly at him, cocked her head to one side, fluttered her eyelashes and pouted her lips as she said, 'Stop blackmailing me, you can't blackmail the blackmailer you know.' She had outmanoeuvred him again and he gave me a little smile. I think Eric rather admired and liked this side of Mollie.

One evening, Gareth, the head coach and under 14s manager at Newcastle Town Football Club, which Jake plays for, telephoned to speak to Lee. Mollie answered the phone and he asked her if he could speak to her daddy, to which Mollie replied, 'Please don't call him Daddy, it's Dad, that is so inappropriate. Oh and by the way my brother says that he doesn't like you because you are moody and mean.' Half an hour later, a frantic Jake ran into the lounge waving his BlackBerry in my face saying, 'What has Mollie been saying to Gareth? Look at this text I've just received.' Jake had received a message from his head coach asking why he thought he was so moody and mean…tee hee!

Talking about Gareth brings me to another story. On one of the rare occasions that Mollie left the home, we went to watch the football team train. Now, Gareth does need to be fairly strict to keep a squad of 18 teenage boys in line. Mollie can be fiercely protective of people whom she likes, so she did not like it when one of Jake's friends, Daniel, was told off by Gareth. She had a bit of a soft spot for Daniel and, at that time, he spent a lot of time round at our house.

She marched up to Gareth like a woman on a mission. Wagging her finger at him, she told him in no uncertain terms, 'You are so mean and bossy, I'm not surprised none of the boys like you, they all hate you. My dad is a far better football manager than you; he should be running this team.'

Both Lee and I were mortified and several apologetic phone calls were made that evening to ensure that Gareth knew that those comments were Mollie's views only and were not views that she had picked up from conversations at home. As Lee was the assistant manager/coach, Gareth was essentially his boss so, while it is very funny looking back, it was rather embarrassing at the time.

One evening I was relaxing with a class of wine and really enjoying some peace and quiet. Following a long and difficult day with Mollie, she had gone to my parents for a sleepover. At 1.00am I received a phone call from my dad who was rather flustered. Mollie was demanding to come home straight away. She was frightened that I was in the house alone and she was concerned over what would happen to me if I fell down the stairs in the night. I would be all alone; who would help me and what if I died?

Mollie was so distraught that my dad and I agreed that he should bring her back home. She was very relieved to see me and that I was alive and well. 'Oh mum, I have been so worried', she said. 'I have been so frightened about you dying because if you died who would look after me?' Charming!

A regular conversation that Mollie has with my parents and with me is to discuss and negotiate what items she would like when we die. So far she has asked my dad for his car and she has asked my mum for her pottery shoe collection, jewellery and her bungalow.

She has also negotiated my mum's collection of flip-flops for me. According to Mollie, I am very low on shoes and I really need and would appreciate my mum's flip-flop collection. How could she refuse? When it comes to my possessions, she has simply requested that when I die can she please have the house?

Finally, never leave your email or Facebook page open if your child with PDA is around. I made this unfortunate mistake when I left an email from 'The' Phil Christie open on my computer. I had not met Phil; at this stage we were simply in the preliminary stages of discussing assessment and so on. A short while later, Phil phoned me to ask if I was okay because he had received an email from me saying, and I quote, 'I hate you, you git'! Luckily it was quickly established whom the culprit was and we could laugh about it.

Similarly, Lee once made the mistake of leaving his Facebook page open. While he was at work, several friends texted him to check if he was feeling alright. 'I'm fine', he replied, 'Why do you ask?' They then informed him that he had been sending out some strange messages, so he checked his account. Mollie had innocently and without malicious intent being writing, 'I'm bored will someone please play with me?' on his timeline. You can understand the confusion that this provoked in his friends.

I could go on for pages but I wouldn't want to bore you. While this behaviour would not be deemed acceptable for a NT child, it is typical for a child with PDA. Although these incidents can be extremely embarrassing, we can't help but smile and secretly enjoy this aspect of her character. The ability to just come out with whatever is on your mind and to do it with such style and panache is very endearing.

A side of Mollie's character that is really nice is that she can be very loving and she really enjoys long cuddles, hugs and snuggling up on the sofa. When you are in her good books she can make you feel like the most loved and special person alive. I suppose that if an individual can show anger to the extreme then it stands to reason that they can also show love to the extreme. She is also extremely loyal to those who she cares about and she will protect and defend you against anyone who she perceives is attacking you.

When Mollie is in a good mood, it takes very little to make her whoop with excitement and laugh like a drain. Her excitement and laughter are contagious and she can make the most mundane of experiences thoroughly enjoyable. She has maintained a very childlike quality, which she will probably continue to have. Although she is only ten years old, there are aspects of her character that remain like that of a much younger child. You would expect to see the games and toys she plays with used by a much younger child.

This is a really sweet and endearing quality. The way that she lets out little squeals and claps her hands in anticipation of a pleasant event – or even during a film when the boy finally gets the girl – shows a much softer and sweeter side to her. Mollie admits that she is a 'hopeless romantic' and her heart just dances and skips when she is watching a feel-good movie.

Mollie's love of practical jokes, her tendency to hide our items and her wonderful ability to completely fabricate the truth or just to tell outright tall stories can also be very amusing. Here are just a few of her stories and practical jokes.

Mollie, in a very matter-of-fact way, told a lady at swimming that she had just returned from a year in the States and that her social worker had a mechanical leg. The lady appeared to fall for this hook, line and sinker.

A few years ago on holiday Mollie spent several days pretending to be a twin to other children. The effort that she put into this role play was definitely to be admired. She would frequently run into the caravan and change her clothes and hairstyle and then re-emerge outside with a different name and persona. Her twin was named Corinne and she would explain to the other children a variety of excuses and reasons as to why the twins were never seen at the same time.

During a trip to our local park, Mollie told another child that her boyfriend was a mass murderer currently spending time in jail. Unfortunately this did get a little bit stressful because Mollie became increasingly anxious and stressed when the other child found this hard to believe. She then became increasingly agitated with me during our journey home, because I wouldn't agree with her that she did indeed have a boyfriend who was a murderer.

She informed her school teachers that we had buried our family dog at 3.00am, which was why she was so tired at school. She must have been rather plausible because they went along with the story not quite sure what to believe. They had to ask me if I could confirm the story because they didn't know if they should be going with the flow of the story and offering their condolences.

My neighbour was stunned to hear that Mollie had been chewing the same piece of chewing gum for ten years. As Mollie was only eight years old at the time, this did seem highly unlikely to be true. Mollie claimed that she had set the new world record for chewing gum!

When Jake had friends to sleep over they made the big mistake of annoying Mollie. Because she was going through a nocturnal phase she easily stayed awake and waited for them to fall asleep. She then crept in and discreetly placed chocolate bars on the pillow and on the bare back of Jake's sleeping friend. A few hours later she quietly chuckled in her bedroom while she listened to the pandemonium breaking out in her brother's bedroom. The poor lad had woken up, confused and covered in melted chocolate, convinced that he must have been sick in his sleep. Fortunately he is a lovely lad with a fabulous sense of humour.

Another time when Jake had a group of friends over from his football team, they again made the mistake of upsetting Mollie. When the group got up to leave the room, they discovered that they were trapped. Mollie had rather ingeniously devised a wonderful system of ropes and knots securing the door to the banister. When the boys tried to open the door into the room, it wouldn't budge, as it was firmly secured by ropes to the banister.

Individuals with PDA are often referred to as Jekyll and Hyde, but it can become easy to concentrate on the Mr Hyde side of their characters and forget to mention the Dr Jekyll side too. It is there, and in the correct environment Dr Jekyll can become the more dominant alter ego.

25

An Interview with Mollie

This is an interview that Mollie gave for one of her guest posts on my blog. She gave me this interview and permission to post it on my blog in the months prior to her going out and dipping her toes back in the outside world.

So, hi I'm Mollie and this is my first article. My mum is going to interview me now, so here it goes.

How does it make you feel if you are asked or told to do something?

It doesn't really feel anything, I don't know that I am avoiding it; it is an instinct to avoid the demand. It's just how I am.

How do you feel if someone tries to make you do something right now and not in your own time?

My stomach goes in knots and I feel anxious like they are yelling at me. I get a bit scared, but I don't show it. If you are going down a big ride it's scary and that is how I feel if someone gives me a direct demand. I can react differently each time and I never know how I will react.

What caused you to have huge meltdowns?

If you are a baby and you want something you would cry and shout until you get it. It is a bit like that; one reason for a meltdown is to get something.

Another reason is if you have a brother and he is getting all of the attention and you think that your parents love him more than you then you will do what you need to get attention. Even if it means being told off, some attention is better than no attention.

If you are so angry, it isn't like normal people, you can't keep it inside, you can't calm down, you have to punch or kick something and you have to release your rage through your arms and legs. People telling me what to do or yelling at me makes me angry. It's like Pompeii all over again except the volcano doesn't stop erupting. My family are the Pompeians and I am the volcano. I can erupt anyplace and anywhere if they make one wrong step – bang!!!

Why don't you have meltdowns anymore?

I don't know why. I don't think that I have changed; I think that you have changed. My environment is different now because I don't go to school and so I feel calmer. I am teaching myself things so I don't need to be taught because I can find things out for myself.

I feel that because I'm at home I feel a lot safer and my nerves are down. My anxiety liquid has also helped to calm my nerves. Also letting me do my own thing and you and Dad not making me stick to lots of your rules or your boundaries helps me to feel calm and in control.

Do you feel bad if you hit or shout at someone?

If I hit someone I feel bad a second later and so I run off. I'm terrified and hope that they won't see me or know that it was me. I'm scared that they won't forgive me or forget what I have done. I do feel regret, anxious and scared after a meltdown and that I need to move away and find new friends because I will have lost those. That is why I could never go back to school after I had a meltdown and was restrained by the teachers.

Why do you think that some stuff isn't rude?

I see people like teenagers and adults say stuff and I want to fit in and so I say that without realising that it's wrong because they laugh at swear words. I'm like – I've heard loads of people say that so why is it wrong? – my mum will tell me that it's wrong.

Because I've got a good memory I remember the words and use them when I am angry. Sometimes I try to make it funny and my friend always laughs at that stuff but I can't tell my mum any of that. Sometimes when I swear I don't care because I get angry but when I see them upset I do feel the tiniest bit of remorse.

Do punishments and boundaries work to make you behave differently?

No, punishments and boundaries don't work because they make me mad instead. Also punishments can make me feel scared and stressed out. I'm not a doctor and so I don't always know why things do or don't work.

Why do you tell lies or make up stories?

Lies about my life and my family are to make me seem more interesting, so I may tell someone that my family and I have been on the biggest rollercoaster in the world. I say things like this so that people will be interested in me and like me.

Other lies, like for example saying, 'Jake, someone has run over Rosebud' (Rosebud is my dog), I would say because I think it is funny to see the reaction. I just think it is funny and I don't naturally think how I have made that person feel.

How do you feel about having PDA – are you happy?

Sometimes I'm not happy but sometimes I am happy because having PDA makes me special. Sometimes I feel that having PDA really messes up my life – people can look at me weird and think that I am weird but I'm not. I am getting used to it and starting to feel more comfortable and confident about myself.

Why do you always interrupt people?

So, my mum keeps asking me this same question. Why do I interrupt people's conversations? Well that's a hard one, but I think it's because I feel like whoever is talking gets all of the attention. So I try to interrupt so that I get the attention, so that's that.

What tip would you give to all those parents out there?

I don't know if it's just me but when my mum ask me questions, like, 'How do you feel when I tell you what to do?', it annoys me and makes me anxious, so that's one tip.

When people talk loud at you how does that make you feel?

I don't know why but when people talk loud its sounds like they are shouting at me and when people do shout it's like a cold vibe goes down me and my nerves go dead bad.

Why do you have to be in control at all times?

I don't have any friends but when I do I have to be in control. I always think if you want something done you've got to do it yourself. So I wish that they were dolls so I could play with them but then I realise that they are not dolls, so that's why.

I also like to be in charge so that I can control my environment. I feel really embarrassed and upset if someone says the wrong thing to me like, 'Don't do that,' or gives me an instruction that I'm not expecting. If I'm in control there is less chance of this happening because I am in charge of them. I like surprises that are good ones but I don't like being surprised by someone else, including other kids, telling me what to do or what to play.

How do you cope with having a brother?

I don't know if this is just me but when my brother's friends are over I have to play and follow them around because I'm jealous that I don't have friends, so I tried to take his. But there is one problem, my brother and his friends are five years older than me.

Why did you stop going out?

I stopped going out because I was scared that I was going to do something stupid in front of loads of people. I feel dead panicky, just panicky.

Why do you steal other people's stuff?

A successful steal used to give me a great adrenaline rush. I would steal loads of stuff and hide it and enjoy watching people look for their stuff. I don't do it anymore, so don't worry if your kids do because they will probably grow out of it.

What are the really positive things about you?

I am very funny; sometimes I say things that make people laugh without meaning to. I am very lively and I have a great imagination. I am extremely clever with a high IQ meaning that I can solve visual problems really easily. I am very creative and really good at art. Oh and I'm a brilliant actress, how do you think I lie so well and fool others into believing my stories? I guess that I am a little bit mischievous because I really love playing pranks and practical jokes.

How can Mum and Dad help you to be the best and the happiest that you can be?

Just carry on with how things are now. No discipline, rules, punishments or anything like that because it makes me more angry. Mum's and Dad's need to be patient, for example don't tell me to brush my teeth NOW! Instead leave the toothbrush on the side and leave it for me to decide when to brush my teeth. Parents need to be fun and exciting so that if I slip up or do something wrong you need to stay calm and say it's alright. Make sure that I am in a safe environment.

Why do you love watching Netflix and the same films over and over again?

Real life can be so boring – there are no witches, warlocks, werewolves, vampires or anything like that in real life. I like watching these shows and pretending that I'm kind of in them and that this is my life. I don't feel like I really fit in with this world and so I like those shows because I feel more normal because werewolves and vampires don't fit in either so they're a bit like me.

Kids with PDA aren't bad, their brains may be wired up different but they aren't that different. We all talk, walk, sneeze and get colds just like everyone else. Don't try and make them be good with treats, prizes or punishments. We need to be treated with respect; we need to be treated like adults because we think more like adults than kids. Try to accept us as different rather than try to make us, what others think of as, normal.

(Mollie Ann Sherwin 2014)

26

Our Current Situation and My Hopes for the Future

It is now July 2014 and Mollie is ten years old. It has been just over one year since we finally ended our pursuit of formal education. During that year Mollie and I have been on a gradual journey of repair, recuperation and awareness. She has been able to educate me and to offer me more and more insight into her world – her fears, her views, her interpretations and her difficulties. I hope that with that insight I have been able to truly, understand, empathise and provide her with better support and the correct environment.

Mollie *can't* simply change in order to fit in and to be able to successfully navigate the NT world. If that was possible I am sure that she would do it in a heartbeat. It is simply a case of *can't* rather than *won't*, which is so vital to understand. Take a fish out of water and it will flap about on the riverside gasping for oxygen. The outside world is Mollie's riverside and the artificial environment that we have created for her at home is her river. Within the river she can swim, be free and be herself.

We hope that with help and support she will gradually be able to last for longer periods of time on the riverbank before the need for oxygen forces her back into the safety of the river. We also hope that we can encourage more people occasionally to leave the comfort of the riverbank, which is the environment within which they flourish, and to test out the waters in the river, gradually building up their tolerance to cope in Mollie's environment.

Mollie is far happier at the moment and she has been restored to the confident, bouncy little girl who I thought I had lost forever. However, if I said that life was easy and that everything was plain sailing, I would be lying.

Mollie is still extremely complex and requires the most careful and delicate of handling in order to continue with the positive achievements that we have made. Achievements have also come at a cost and that cost has been to say goodbye to the life that I had previously imagined for myself and for my family.

I now have to live a completely alternative lifestyle from the one that I had envisaged. I have, at times, felt that I had to completely sacrifice my own life and my own happiness in order to facilitate what Mollie needs. It is physically and mentally exhausting, not to mention lonely and isolating, to support her needs and provide her with an environment within which she can flourish.

Everything that comes naturally to me and everything that I have learned during my 43 years on this planet with regard to social interaction and communication is absolutely useless for communicating with Mollie. It is extremely challenging to continually have to interact and communicate with another individual in a way that is totally unnatural and foreign to one's own instincts.

At times, I have felt very resentful, not towards Mollie but towards PDA. I have grieved for the life that I feel that PDA has taken away from me and from my daughter. I am now in the process of adjusting to and accepting where we are now and where the future will take us. Our family as a whole is a happier and calmer place to be, so no matter how hard this new existence is to adjust to, it is the only choice. I am gradually getting used to and focusing on the positives rather than the negatives as we continue on our very alternative journey through life.

I am finding happiness and contentment in my new life and I am, finally, really letting go of my old life. I feel that this life is my destiny and that this is the path that I was meant to walk. My wonderful daughter was given to me so that we could learn, grow and educate those around us and eventually to help others like 'her' together. We are a team, a unit, Mollie and I against the world, and at times that really is how we have felt.

Although I do not intend to pursue any further school placements, I wouldn't completely rule out a return to formal education if it is something that I feel would, in the future, be beneficial for Mollie. Until such time, Mollie shall continue to be educated at home by simply learning through life.

Each day we do what Mollie wants within the parameters of what I can realistically achieve. She may spend the day on the computer and watching Netflix or she may want to play all day, go for a walk, do arts and crafts or bake. More recently we have also enjoyed trips to the cinema and bowling. Over the last few months, she has tentatively been going out to play in the street with other children.

There are still times when her need for total control and her inability to occupy herself for more than ten seconds resurfaces. These periods are really difficult because that need for control and constant interaction can start at 8.00am and continue until midnight at the earliest. Even though this load is shared between my husband and I and our support network, it really can get to be too much.

I do reach my limits and, even though it may upset her, I have to remind Mollie that I am neither a robot nor a plaything and I just can't keep up with such an intense desire for her to be entertained by me or cope with the extreme control that she may be exerting over me. I may need to stay firm during these periods in order to preserve my sanity and simply absorb any abuse that may come my way. Due to our overall lifestyle and the limited demands placed on her, the fallout from standing my ground no longer appears to explode with quite the intensity that it used to.

Ann, our personal assistant funded for seven hours a week by social services via direct payments, is only in her twenties and really fills the void of a peer of Mollie's own age. Ann plays with Mollie on her level and Mollie has started to chat and banter with Ann in a way that she would with a peer.

Such conversations obviously aren't for Mum's ears; I am far too old! Mollie also has social interactions with her dad, brother, aunt and uncle and she is very close to her maternal grandparents. So she does experience very positive social interaction with people who understand, love and can accommodate her. This is a small and limited group but we are hopeful that in time this may expand to a few more people. For now this group is the ideal for Mollie and provides her with what she needs without spiking anxiety levels or making her feel as if she is a failure.

Providing Mollie with the correct support and strategies personally tailored to her individual personality and needs has brought us outstanding results. There are almost no violent meltdowns, limited verbal outbursts and while her behaviour is still complex to manage, it is no longer as challenging. With full control over her own life, within our minimal boundaries and parameters, she really doesn't maliciously do anything wrong or behave in a naughty way.

She still behaves in a PDA fashion, because that is who she is, so it is important to establish that PDA behaviours are not naughty behaviours that need stamping out, they simply need accommodating. She isn't breaking windows, running off, ruining our furniture with graffiti or breaking the law. So we simply accept that although she can't follow direct demands or behave as we would traditionally expect a child to behave, that is okay. Because for a child with PDA, her behaviour could probably be described as exceptional and that is the yardstick with which we need to measure her.

Another huge improvement for us is that Mollie has started, only when she is at her most relaxed, to communicate verbally how she feels and perceives the world through her eyes. The quality of the information that she delivers is astounding and is invaluable to further my understanding of her. Children with PDA generally find it very difficult to verbalise their feelings and this is no different for Mollie. Previously internal feelings were simply expressed through her behaviour. To a large degree this is still the case, but verbal explanations are also increasingly being used for her to express herself either during or after an event.

Another important step forward for me is the revelation that I need to 'roll with it' when it comes to Mollie's cycles of behaviour. Instead of swimming upstream and trying to alter sleeping patterns, encourage more interaction and less screen time, reduce her need for attention when it reaches suffocating and overbearing levels or continually pushing for her to engage more with the outside world, I have decided to take a step back.

I have discovered that everything with Mollie appears to run in cycles and that these cycles will naturally come to an end and alternate with each other. So I will no longer question my parenting skills or what else I should be doing the next time she turns night into day. Instead I will simply 'roll with it', safe in the knowledge that this cycle will eventually run its course and be replaced with a more traditional sleep cycle.

Weeks of Mollie being engrossed in repetitive TV-series watching and screen time will eventually be replaced with weeks of Mollie being completely unable to occupy herself, during which times she will demand complete and utter one-on-one attention. However, as previously stated, we can reach extremes when this situation may no longer be tolerable, so in order to preserve my own sanity I may have to try and rein the need for attention and control in. The cycles continue to revolve and I am gradually getting used to 'rolling with it' rather than worrying.

However, despite all of my best efforts, I am only human. I have days when I feel low and sad, and I experience regular bouts of depression and anxiety. The years of abuse from Mollie coupled, with the years of battling to have her condition understood and her needs met, have left my nervous system permanently damaged. I now take fluoxetine and this is hugely beneficial in keeping my nervous system on a more even keel.

I have days when my energy and patience is low. On these days, all of my own experiences and strategies may completely fly out of the window. I will do everything wrong from a PDA point of view and I may be more prone to snapping or shouting. When I have days like these, I need to forgive myself and not give myself a hard time for not being able to be the 'perfect PDA parent' all of the time. When I know that I have had a bad day, managed Mollie wrongly or been a general pain in the bum I do apologise to Mollie so that she knows that the fault is with me and not her. She has become very forgiving of me during these days and often says, 'It's okay, don't worry about it.' The next day is a new day and we start afresh from there.

In a similar fashion, Mollie has off days too when, regardless of how I try to parent her, she can still be a very prickly and angry customer. When Mollie has these moments she will often apologise too and she may confess that she is short-tempered because she is feeling stressed and so on. Of course, there are other times when she will apologise but remind me that it was my fault that she lost her temper, but that's PDA for you. I hope that in time, and with careful guidance, I will be able to help her to take responsibility for her own actions. I guess that what I am trying to emphasise here is that none of us are perfect, so the important part is how we resolve and move on from disputes or difficult days rather than the fact that we will inevitably continue to experience them.

When it comes to Mollie's future, I would rather be realistic and accept that she will probably need help and support throughout her life. If she doesn't then great but, if I'm being honest, this is something that I feel I need to prepare for. I don't feel that she will ever be able to work or financially support herself. I am not trying to be negative, and if she does achieve these things it would be amazing, but I have to be realistic.

That being said, Mollie shall always be actively encouraged to achieve anything that she feels is possible. We have a reasonably sized home and a large double garage. Our plan, should Mollie wish, is to convert part of our home into a self-contained living area for her. This will give her independence and her own space while still having us on hand to take care of her and to meet her needs.

I am hopeful that she will be able to find happiness, her place in the world and a life partner who can accept and help her. If she does achieve this, then I will be ecstatic and I can honestly say that my dreams will have become a reality.

With growing awareness, my wonderful and supportive family, the PDA community and the small army of professionals driving PDA recognition forward, the future for Mollie and for those who follow in her footsteps should be a much brighter one than for those who preceded her.

Appendix 1

A Complete Profile of Mollie's Behaviours and Traits

All children with PDA will be unique. However, I have listed all of the unusual characteristics that Mollie displays, which may be helpful in providing a more complete picture of how the personality and traits of a child with PDA may present. I have categorised them by the difficulties associated with ASD to show how this profile slots into an atypical ASD profile but with the additional unique features that identify her as specifically, and more accurately, belonging to the PDA subgroup.

Social understanding and imagination

- Mollie does not appear to understand the natural social pecking order. She does not seem to see herself as a child or understand her natural place in society or how to behave in relation to those around her.

- Mollie can have great difficulty in adjusting her behaviour to different social contexts, for example waiting quietly at the doctor's, behaving appropriately in shops, adjusting her behaviour for adults, following demands at school and so on.

- Mollie can be very overfamiliar with those around her, for example quickly sitting on a person's knee or wanting a cuddle from someone who she has only just met or with a person where this would be seen as inappropriate, such as a teacher.

- Mollie may appear to have better empathy than other children on the spectrum but this can seem to be on an intellectual level rather than an emotional one. She can use her empathy skills to manipulate, control and avoid situations but often appears to have little understanding of the emotional effect that her actions may have on others.

- Mollie's apparent difficulty seeing things from another person's perspective at an emotional level can lead to problems in resolving conflict.

- Mollie doesn't appear to understand fully or to be able to empathise with how her words may hurt someone at an emotional level, for example she may openly tell someone if she thinks that they are fat or ugly or inappropriately laugh at something that others would not find funny. Mollie can take delight in embarrassing somebody else.

- Mollie can love playing practical jokes but she doesn't appear to understand naturally the boundaries of when a joke is going too far or whether the recipient of the joke will find it funny. If the recipient is upset by the joke Mollie can still find it funny.

- Mollie can become heavily involved in role play and the lines of imagination and reality can be blurred.

- Stealing objects from around the home and hiding them started when Mollie was about three years old. She wouldn't necessarily steal desirable objects, so it was more about the fun and humour of the act and enjoying seeing people's reactions than actually acquiring a certain possession.

- She will often talk to us through a soft toy, and cuddly toys have become a major part of Mollie's life.

- Mollie often tells lies, tales of fantasy and made-up stories either about herself or others, but she may appear confused and/or upset if these stories are not believed or not received well when others realise that they are untrue. She will do this for fun or to make herself appear more interesting to others. She feels that she needs to be more interesting to other people or they will find her dull and boring.

Social interaction

- When Mollie does not feel in complete control of her immediate environment and the people in it, she can become very verbally and physically aggressive due to high anxiety.

- She interacts with other people by controlling and directing everyone, which is reminiscent of a director directing a play.

- Her body language and facial expression often appear to be over the top, acted, mimicked or melodramatic, possibly due to Mollie's huge capacity to role play and mimic what she sees those around her doing, especially on TV.

- Mollie can try to isolate a particular child from the rest of the class/group in order to try to maintain that friendship by reducing the possibility of other children from taking her/him away from her.

- Mollie appears to cope much better in a one-on-one social situation and struggles to an even higher degree in group situations. This may further explain the need for her to have one close friend with whom she can interact on a one-on-one level.

- Mollie can appear to interact with other individuals as if they are simply objects or playthings that are there for her amusement. People can appear to be moved and organised like chess pieces on a chessboard.

- Mollie does appear to have better eye contact than other children on the autism spectrum.

- Mollie can appear to be very social and she can role play appropriate behaviours, but the ability to sustain this role play can vary.

- Once the novelty of a new friend or situation wears off, Mollie can become more comfortable and less able to maintain the role play of the 'perfect child'. This is when the difficulties that she experiences and her natural behaviours become more obvious to others.

- Ultimately, Mollie, due to her need to be in control, has found it increasingly difficult to maintain a healthy relationship with peers and following repeated failures and low self-esteem she has become very reclusive.

- Other children may actively avoid Mollie, feeling frightened or confused by her controlling and unpredictable behaviour.

- Mollie can become the object of ridicule and bullying by other children who confuse her difficulties with those of simply being a bossy, naughty child. They can learn which buttons to push in order to prompt an outburst from her.

- Mollie can become so needy for a friend that she herself may be at risk of being manipulated by other children who recognise this weakness and utilise it for their own purposes.

- Increasing awareness of her difficulties and the anxiety that socialising causes have resulted in Mollie failing to initiate any social interaction as she has grown older.

- She is highly competitive and she must win at all costs. Cheating and conning others in order to win are almost seen as part of the fun by Mollie.

- Extreme jealousy became a very strong and obvious trait from very early childhood. Mollie has to be the centre of attention and even as a toddler she would physically intervene to move me away from Jake if he was getting any attention from me.

Social communication

- Mollie appears to misunderstand tone of voice and the speaker's intention, often feeling that she is being told off, shouted at, purposefully embarrassed or ordered/bossed about.

- Mollie tries to dominate both her own conversations and those of others with the use of many strategies, such as constantly interrupting the flow of conversations, not allowing anyone else to speak, bombarding others with repetitive questions, refusing to respond to questions that are asked of her or responding by switching the conversation to a different topic. It can often appear that conversation is simply a tool that is used to avoid the demands of others or to dominate and control their actions.

- Mollie can often speak in quite complex sentences and the context of the language can seem bizarre for a child of her age. Language may be copied or imitated from adults, other children or from the media but may not necessarily be understood by Mollie.

- Mollie can pronounce certain words in her own unique way, for example saying 'defore' instead of 'before' or 'smarshmellows' instead of 'marshmallows'.

- Mollie can have difficulty in understanding sarcasm and humour, sometimes taking comments literally.

- Verbal communication has not been a vehicle that Mollie has used to express her thoughts, fears or needs, which have mainly been expressed through behaviour.

Obsessions

- Mollie can become obsessed with a particular person, from either a love or a hate perspective.

- At times Mollie can become obsessed with human contact and during these times she may simply be unable to be in her own company. This can become very suffocating and stressful for the main carer, because Mollie will literally crave every minute of your attention 24/7.

- The need to control and avoid demands could be seen as an obsessive behaviour and she does impose this behaviour on others.

- She can repeatedly watch the same film or TV series time after time and/or need to watch a whole series all the way through.

- Mollie may become obsessed with a particular toy or style of play, such as Barbie, and that may become the only game that she plays.

- Mollie can often seem to have become fixated on a particular soft toy, which may then take on a whole persona of its own.

- Mollie can become obsessed with particular computer or Xbox games, needing to play them for hours on end.

- Mollie can become obsessed with purchasing certain items. A desired item can become all-consuming and the need to have it does not dissipate until the item has been purchased.

- She loves to collect things and can become obsessed with obtaining everything and anything to do with her latest obsession, such as the full infantry of Moshi Monsters merchandise or everything to do with Barbie, Power Rangers etc. Sometimes this love of collecting may extend to more unusual items, for example marbles, rocks and various trinkets.

- A recently acquired obsession is the need to know and see people's reactions to certain events. She is continually pestering me to act out my own reactions to something that has recently happened and to explain how I felt or to act out another person's reactions to a particular incident.

Repetitive routines and the need for sameness

- Many of her behaviours appear to run in cycles, for example weeks of refusing to sleep at nights can be replaced by weeks of insisting on being, and becoming anxious if she isn't, in bed for the correct time. Mollie's whole life can appear to be a system of routines that revolve around a repetitive cycle.

- Mollie has had periods when she developed repetitive skin picking and facial and verbal tics.

- Mollie can become greatly distressed if her belongings are moved or tidied away. Things may need to be left in the position that she left them.

- Mollie has a very limited repertoire for food, often insisting on eating the same things again and again.

- The need to control and avoid demands could be seen as a repetitive behaviour and she does impose this behaviour on others.

- Mollie has a tendency for repetitive questioning especially if she is trying to control a situation.

- Mollie does not like routine that is imposed on her by others but she has developed a need to adhere to her own routine and will impose this routine on others. Using novelty can sometimes be successful in helping her to engage in an activity that may not be part of her usual routine.

- Mollie has developed a routine involving people. Only certain people can perform certain tasks, for example I wake her up and do the morning routine, Dad does the bedtime routine, I play arts and crafts, Dad plays computer games, her personal assistant plays Barbie and so on, and no one can ever switch roles.

- She may repetitively colour in picture after picture of her latest focus of interest.

- Sometimes she has slightly more unusual interests, like tying things up with intricate knots, cutting up yoghurt pots, making glass after glass of coloured water etc.

- Play can be imaginative but it will often also be repetitive. Mollie will often appear to be the scriptwriter and the director, and the other child is simply there to obey Mollie's demands rather than to contribute actively.

Sensory issues

- Mollie does have sensory issues and she has been diagnosed as having sensory processing disorder by an occupational therapist.

Frequently Asked Questions
by Phil Christie and Ruth Fidler

Below are a number of questions that Jane Sherwin has found to be commonly asked by parents of children with PDA. The responses to these questions have been given by Phil Christie and Ruth Fidler. Most of these appear in one form or another on the websites, or literature of the PDA society or the Elizabeth Newson Centre. They may also have been given in response to questions asked in online forums.

QUESTIONS ABOUT DIAGNOSIS

* **Is PDA part of the autism spectrum and how does it differ from other conditions that are described within the spectrum such as autism?**

The term Pathological Demand Avoidance syndrome (PDA) was first used by Professor Elizabeth Newson in the 1980's in a series of clinical descriptions, small-scale research articles, informal publications and lecture presentations. It wasn't, though, until 2003 that the first article on PDA appeared in a peer-reviewed journal (*Archives of Disease in Childhood*), in which Newson proposed that PDA be recognised as 'a separate entity within the pervasive developmental disorders'.

At that time both of the diagnostic manuals (DSM and ICD) used Pervasive Developmental Disorder (PDD) as the umbrella term under which autism and Asperger syndrome were placed. One of the reasons that PDA has become widely recognised as part of the autism spectrum is that the term Autism Spectrum Disorder (ASD) itself became to mean the same as PDD and replaced it in everyday language. This was acknowledged by the National Autism Plan for Children in 2003 and, later, the NICE guidelines on autism diagnosis.

Over the last few years there has been a huge upsurge in interest in PDA due to a strong, and continued, sense of recognition amongst parents and others on reading the clinical descriptions and accounts of PDA. Along with this there has come a realisation, particularly amongst educationalists, that children and young people who fit the PDA profile require a modified and adapted approach to teaching and learning. More and more professionals feel that PDA is best regarded as being part of the autism spectrum.

In order for there to be a wider endorsement of PDA within diagnostic services and recognition within the manuals a stronger research base is needed. Professor Francesca Happé (Director of the MRC at the Institute of Psychiatry) when speaking at the first NAS/NORSACA conference in 2011, talked about the cogency of the clinical descriptions and the sense of recognition of this profile amongst parents and many professionals, but also of the paucity of research evidence. The project undertaken by the IoP has set out to start addressing this and two more papers have now appeared in peer reviewed journals. More details about this research and references can be found at: https://sites.google.com/site/lizonions/ moreinfoaboutresearch.

One paper, published in the *Journal of Child Psychology and Psychiatry*, describes the development of the Extreme Demand Avoidance Questionnaire (EDA-Q) to quantify the behaviours within the PDA profile and this shows great potential to assist in identification and future research. This will lead us to better understand which behaviours or features are especially characteristic of children with PDA and which are shared with other children on the autism spectrum.

❖ **Is it possible for someone to have a dual diagnosis of autism and PDA or Asperger syndrome and PDA and, therefore have two diagnoses?**

In the context of the debate described in answer to the first question, PDA is best understood as being part of the autism spectrum. Within the spectrum some individuals clearly present with a very distinct profile of PDA, or Asperger syndrome, while others share characteristics of both. Some people though seem to show more of an 'overlapping presentation'. This is a better way of understanding it than suggesting that they have two distinct conditions.

❖ **What are the differences between PDA, ODD and Attachment Disorder?**

It is inevitably the case that when conditions are defined by what are essentially lists of behavioural features there will be interconnections and overlaps. Aspects of both of these conditions can present in a similar way to those features that make up the profile of PDA. There is also the possibility of the co-existence or 'co-morbidity' of different conditions and where this is the case the presentation is especially complex.

ODD, Oppositional Defiant Disorder, itself often exists alongside ADHD, and is characterised by persistent 'negative, hostile and defiant behaviour' towards authority. There are obvious similarities here with the demand avoidant behaviour of children with PDA. PDA, though, is made up of more than this, the avoidance and need to control is rooted in anxiety and alongside genuine difficulties in social understanding, which is why it is seen as part of the autism spectrum. This isn't the case with descriptions of ODD. A small project, supervised by Elizabeth Newson, compared a group of children with ODD and those with a diagnosis of PDA and found that the children with PDA used a much wider range of avoidance strategies, including a degree of social manipulation. The children described as having ODD tended to refuse and be oppositional but not use the range of other strategies. Many children with ODD and their families are said to be helped by positive parenting courses, which is less often the case with children with PDA.

Attachment disorder, or Reactive Attachment Disorder as described in the diagnostic manuals, has its own debates about how it is best defined. RAD describes a group of children who show 'inhibited, emotionally withdrawn behaviour' and also 'a persistent social or emotional disturbance'. The criteria, though, also include patterns of 'extremes of insufficient care' and are not judged to meet the criteria for autism spectrum disorder. Some professionals prefer to use the term attachment disorder or attachment problems, recognising that attachment is part of a continuum. There is though little research in this area. When children have experienced a very difficult early life, or suffered serious abuse or trauma the presenting problems can appear similar to those of children on the autism spectrum, including those who fit the profile for PDA. One attempt to tease out some of these overlaps and differences was made in producing the Coventry Grid (see: www.aettraininghubs. org.uk/wp-content/uploads/2012/05/5.4-Moran-paper-attachment.pdf).

These areas of overlap, and the potential for behavioural profiles being interpreted in different ways, underlines the importance of a detailed and comprehensive assessment being carried out by experienced practitioners. Assessments should include the taking of a detailed developmental history, as it is vital to know not just how a child presents now but how they developed up until now. This is not always easy with an older child, or a child who grew up in adverse circumstances, as that information might be hard to come by. Assessments should also include detailed observation of the child looking at all areas of development, information about how they behave in a range of different situations, the views of other professionals and consideration of other relevant factors and circumstances, such as their health and family relationships.

QUESTIONS ABOUT BEHAVIOUR

❖ **My child often makes up stories and lies, is this common?**

It is common for children and young people with PDA to become so involved in role-play and pretend that they blur the edges between reality and fantasy.

Sometimes this means that they can truly convince themselves that something really did or didn't happen which can obviously come across to the other people they live or work with as if it is a lie. In this case it is not usually done with intent. On the other hand, making up stories can also be quite an effective way of getting attention, and sticking to that story can be an effective way of sidestepping any responsibility or of passing the blame for a situation. These are other possible explanations for a 'lie'. It should not be forgotten that these children and young people have difficulty understanding the social and emotional consequences of their own words and actions, that they may enjoy the shock factor of fabricated stories and that they may have trouble controlling their impulses. These factors make it more likely that they don't see the wider picture of the damage to relationships or to everyday situations if they say things that are not true. Sometimes it is not worth a head to head 'Yes you did!' 'No I didn't!' argument but it is reasonable to talk about how your perception or understanding of a situation differs form theirs. In a calmer moment it will be important to explain and try to improve their understanding of the consequences and risks of telling stories or lies.

* **My child often takes other people's possessions and hides them, is this common?**

Children and young people with PDA tend to be self-centred in their thinking and have genuine difficulty connecting emotionally with the feelings of other people. Hiding or stealing something may be explained simply as the fact that they want the item themselves and in the context of having difficulty empathising with the person they have taken it from, as well as issues regarding taking responsibility for their own actions, there is little to prevent them doing so. However they are often very good at predicting how certain other people may react, so sometimes doing so may be in order to set someone else up or to provoke another person or to punish them. It is important to understand how the child was interpreting the situation at the time. It is also important to educate them about the social, emotional and ultimately legal consequences of stealing.

❖ **When my child gets really angry how can I tell if they are having a meltdown or if they just want their own way, like any other child?**

Individuals with PDA are precisely that, individuals. Therefore they have their own unique personality, which means they will have differing attitudes and characteristics. Some children and young people with PDA may just be on the edge of cheekiness, whereas others will inevitably be more actively mischievous or defiant. These are ordinary features of lots of children of course. The difference between recognising them simply wanting their own and from having a meltdown, is usually understood by their degree of anxiety and awareness. Of course you have to know the child well to be able to make these judgments. Essentially, children and young people are most probably having a meltdown if they are beyond reason, if they are very anxious or even panicking, if they seem unaware of their actions, if they are unable to extract themselves form this mood or if they have difficulty recalling what happened.

❖ **Why is my child so different in the way they behave at different times or in different places? She often seems much better with other people than when she is with me.**

Children with PDA are quite often variable in the way that they behave and this is often to do with their level of anxiety and fluctuating ability to control or regulate their emotions. At times when their anxiety is low they are calmer and more tolerant and, conversely, when it is high they are more irritable and resistant. Some children's anxiety level goes up and down frequently throughout the day and is influenced by a whole range of factors. This can make them very unpredictable and those around them often say that 'it's like walking on eggshells'.

Families frequently report that their children are very different at home than they are at school. Sometimes, like other children on the autism spectrum, their behaviour is different in different contexts e.g. children may eat certain foods at grandparents but not at home. For children and young people with PDA it is common that many aspects of their behaviour are notably different not only in various settings but also with different people. Behaviour is not surprisingly most difficult when under stress. It is not unusual for children and young people to 'hold it together' and contain their emotions at school (maybe where they feel more exposed or are playing a role) and to vent their feelings when they get home (where they may feel more at liberty to do so). One of the huge challenges for families is that this variability can make their child difficult to manage in ways that other people do not see, do not understand, or in some instances believe. Professionals who have a good understanding of the nature of PDA will recognise that this can be a particular issue for families.

❖ **My child is displaying inappropriate sexualised behaviour at a young age, is this part of PDA?**

Children and young people with PDA are sometimes reported as displaying sexualised behaviour, particularly girls. There may be a number of reasons that contribute to this and dealing with it is certainly not easy for parents or professionals. Reasons for this could include a lack of social understanding and therefore a lack of social inhibition; sensory processing and modulating differences; a drive to use shocking behaviour (sexualised behaviour is an especially effective way of distracting people and of avoiding demands); seeking positive relationships with others by wanting to please them without knowing how to handle a mature intimate relationship; issues regarding impulse control alongside a poor understanding the consequences of their behaviour. Lots of children and young people experiment with adult type of behaviour but typically developing children are usually better at making judgments that keep them safe and protected. The factors outlined above make some children and young people with PDA very vulnerable.

QUESTIONS ABOUT GROWING UP

❖ **Will my child grow out of their condition? Will they ever be able to live an independent life or will they continue to need care and support as an adult?**

The National Autistic Society on their web site, describes autism as 'a lifelong developmental disability' and the same is true for PDA, which is best understood as part of the autism spectrum. A spectrum condition means that, while all people with PDA share certain difficulties, their condition will affect them in different ways and to a different extent

There is a need to gather more information about children with PDA as they grow into adulthood so that we can better understand some of the issues that face them at this time of transition into adulthood.

Elizabeth Newson carried out a survey in 1999, following up a sample of 18 individuals aged 16 and over who had an earlier diagnosis of PDA. She found that the features that characterise the PDA profile were persistent and endured over time. All but one individual was described as still 'obsessively resistant' but seven young people were seen as less avoidant than formerly.

As far as their educational experience and attainments were concerned, unsurprisingly, it was found that a high level of individual support had been essential in maintaining their school placement. Only one participant in the study achieved GCSE standard, although another young person declined participation in the study saying that she was at university abroad following very good support throughout school. In a later, but smaller sample of six, as part of a student research project, the picture was more positive in this respect and three out of the six attained GCSE standard with one of these going on to University.

Many parents have found the information reported in the outcome study as discouraging. It should be remembered though, that the young people included may not have been fully representative of the condition as a whole. As they had already come to the attention of the Elizabeth Newson Centre it is likely that they were mostly those young people with more significant needs. As the study was some while ago it was also at a time when very little was known, or understood, about some of the teaching and management approaches that are proving more effective.

At the same time individuals with PDA and their families are likely to need support throughout their lives. Parents fears for the future mirror those of parents of children with other ASDs, but may be magnified by the variable recognition and understanding of the condition and some of the particular challenges in behaviour that persist for some young people with PDA.

The adult autism strategy issued guidance for local authorities and health bodies on supporting the needs of adults with autism (*Fulfilling and Rewarding lives: The strategy for adults with autism in England*, Department of Health, 2010). This guidance sends a clear message to local councils and health bodies that they must improve training for staff, identification and diagnosis in adults, planning of services and local leadership. It is clearly the intention of this guidance to significantly improve the way that services are delivered for all adults on the autism spectrum. Within this it should also improve some of the experiences and opportunities for people with PDA and underlines the need for the condition to be recognised, identified and understood as being part of the autism spectrum.

❖ **My child can be quite aggressive and violent. Will this get worse as he/she grows older?**

Not all children with PDA show aggression or violence but a proportion do as part of a meltdown when their levels of stress or anxiety get too much. Alternatively this sort of behaviour might have become part of the range of strategies that the child or young person has become to use as part of their avoidance and need to be in control. Typically this comes at the end of an 'escalation' of different strategies, when others have failed. Some children, though, begin to use it as a first response rather than a last resort. If the child or young person is supported and managed well and is helped to understand his or her own emotions better, there is no particular reason that it should get worse as he or she gets older. Indeed many children who are quite explosive when they are younger can learn to control their aggression as they get older. Of course though, as the young person grows older the intensity of any aggressive outbursts might become more severe, even if they are less frequent.

Useful Resources

Websites
Norsaca
www.norsaca.org.uk
Norsaca offers a wide range of services designed to support people affected by autism, including family services, a specialist school – Sutherland House – and outreach and supported living services, as well as residential and day services for young people and adults with autism. They also provide telephone advice and counselling and run specialist training for parents and professionals. They also operate the Elizabeth Newson Centre, which is one of only a few autism-specific diagnostic and assessment centres in the country and the most specialist and experienced centre for diagnosing PDA.

PDA Society
www.pdasociety.org.uk
The PDA Society provides lots of helpful information, contact details for help and advice and a private discussion forum.

The PDA Resource
www.thepdaresource.com
The PDA Resource website, designed and maintained by Graeme Storey, brings together all of the relevant and current information about PDA from across the internet. There is also a

support group page where you can access all of the current PDA Facebook support groups.

Pathological Demand Avoidance Syndrome: An autistic spectrum condition by Neville Starnes

www.youtube.com / user / bluemillicent

Under the name of 'bluemillicent' this is an excellent YouTube channel with lots of vital and informative information for parents from a parent.

The National Autistic Society

www.autism.org.uk

The National Autistic Society is the leading UK charity for people with an ASD and their families. It provides information, support and pioneering services, and campaigns for a better world for people with autism.

Autism Teaching Strategies

www.autismteachingstrategies.com

Autism Teaching Strategies has lots of free downloads, videos and activities for teaching social skills.

Sensory Processing Disorder

www.sensory-processing-disorder.com

Sensory Processing Disorder is an extremely informative site that can tell you everything that you need to know about sensory issues.

Liz O'Nions

https:/ / sites.google.com / site / lizonions

Liz O'Nions is currently a post-doctoral research associate at University College London. The main focus of her PhD research was to understand more about how social processing and empathy are affected in developmental disorders, such as ASDs, and PDA. Liz's PhD supervisors were Professor Francesca Happé and Professor Essi Viding.

MIND

www.mind.org.uk
Mind is a charity that aims to provide help and support and to empower those suffering with mental health issues.

Books

Christie, P., Duncan, M., Healy, Z. and Fidler, R. (2011) *Understanding Pathological Demand Avoidance in Children.* London: Jessica Kingsley Publishers.

Greene, R.W. (2001) *The Explosive Child.* New York, NY: HarperCollins Publishers.

Hurley, E. (ed.) (2014) *Ultraviolet Voices Stories of Women on the Autism Spectrum.* Birmingham: Autism West Midlands.

Biel, L. and Peske, N. (2009) *Raising a Sensory Smart Child: The Definitive Handbook for Helping Your Child with Sensory Processing Issues.* New York, NY: Penguin.

Thomas, A. and Pattison, H. (2009) *How Children Learn at Home.* London: Continuum International Publishing Group.

Peer-reviewed published research

Newson, E., Le Maréchal, K. and David, C. (2003) 'Pathological demand avoidance syndrome: A necessary distinction within the pervasive developmental disorders.' *Archives of Diseases in Childhood 88*, 595–600.

Christie, P. (2007) 'The distinctive clinical and educational needs of children with pathological demand avoidance syndrome, guidelines for good practice.' *Good Autism Practice Journal, May*, 3–11.

Eaton, J. and Banting, R. (2012) 'Adult diagnosis of pathological demand avoidance – subsequent care planning.' *Journal of Learning Disabilities and Offending Behaviour 3*, 3, 150–157.

O'Nions, E., Christie, P., Gould, J., Viding, E. and Happé, F. (2014) 'Development of the 'Extreme Demand Avoidance Questionnaire' (EDA-Q): Preliminary observations on a trait measure for pathological demand avoidance.' *Journal of Child Psychology and Psychiatry 55*, 7, 758–768.

O'Nions, E., Viding, E., Greven, C. U., Ronald, A. and Happé, F. (2013) 'Pathological demand avoidance (PDA): Exploring the behavioural profile.' *Autism: The International Journal of Research and Practice 18*, 5, 538–544.

References

Christie, P., Duncan, M., Healy, Z. and Fidler, R. (2011) *Understanding Pathological Demand Avoidance in Children.* London: Jessica Kingsley Publishers.

Department for Children, School and Families (2007 and 2013) *Elective Home Education Guidelines for Local Authorities.* London: Department for Children, School and Families. Available at www.gov.uk/government/uploads/system/uploads/attachment_data/file/288135/guidelines_for_las_on_elective_home_educationsecondrevisev2_0.pdf, accessed on 3 November 2014.

Eaton, J. and Banting, R. (2012) 'Adult diagnosis of pathological demand avoidance – subsequent care planning.' *Journal of Learning Disabilities and Offending Behaviour 3*, 3, 150–157.

Gould, J. (2011) Pathological Demand Avoidance Conference. London.

National Autistic Society (2009) 'What is PDA?' *Communication,* Winter 2009, 45.

National Autism Standards (2012). *The Distinctive Clinical and Educational Needs of Children with Pathological Demand Avoidance Syndrome: Guidelines for Good Practice.* London: Autism Education Trust. Available at www.aettraininghubs.org.uk/wp-content/uploads/2012/05/5.2-strategies-for-teaching-pupils-with-PDA.pdf, accessed 3 November 2014.

National Initiative for Autism: Screening and Assessment (2003) *National Autism Plan for Children: Plan for the Identification, Assessment, Diagnosis and Access to Early Interventions for Pre-school Children with Autism Spectrum Disorders.* London: National Autistic Society.

National Institute for Health and Care Excellence (2011) *Autism Diagnosis in Children and Young People: Recognition, Referral and Diagnosis of Children and Young People on the Autism Spectrum.* London: Department of Health.

Newson, E. and David, C. (1999) 'Pathological demand avoidance syndrome: What is the outlook?' In P. Shattock and G. Linfoot (eds) *From Research Into Therapy.* Sunderland: University of Sunderland.

Newson, E., Le Maréchal, K. and David, C. (2003) 'Pathological demand avoidance syndrome: A necessary distinction within the pervasive developmental disorders.' *Archives of Diseases in Childhood 88,* 595–600.

O'Nions, E. (2014) *Understanding Thoughts and Responding to Emotions: Exploring Similarities and Differences Between Autism Spectrum Disorders, Conduct Problems with Callous-unemotional Traits, and Pathological Demand Avoidance.* Unpublished doctoral dissertation. London: King's College London.

O'Nions, E., Christie, P., Gould, J., Viding, E. and Happé, F. (2013a) 'Development of the 'Extreme Demand Avoidance Questionnaire' (EDA-Q): Preliminary observations on a trait measure for pathological demand avoidance.' *Journal of Child Psychology and Psychiatry 55,* 7, 758–768.

O'Nions, E., Viding, E., Greven, C. U., Ronald, A. and Happé, F. (2013b) 'Pathological demand avoidance (PDA): Exploring the behavioural profile.' *Autism: The International Journal of Research and Practice 18,* 5, 538–544.

The NHS Commissioning Board (2013) *The Functions of Clinical Commissioning Groups.* Redditch: Commissioning Development Directorate. Available at www.england.nhs. uk/wp-content/uploads/2013/03/a-functions-ccgs.pdf, accessed on 3 November 2014.

Thomas, A. and Pattison, H. (2009) *How Children Learn at Home.* London: Continuum International Publishing Group.